Forty plus Thirty

The Road To Healthy Aging

Michael Stapenhurst

I0441851

Copyright © 2018

All rights reserved. No part of this book may be reproduced or transmitted in any form or by any means, electronic, manual, photocopying, recording, or by any information and retrieval system, without prior written permission of the author.

Disclaimer

The Author has striven to be as accurate and complete as possible in the creation of this book. While all attempts have been made to verify information provided in this publication, the Author assumes no responsibility for errors, omissions, or contrary interpretation of the subject matter herein.

All information in 'Forty plus Thirty' is intended for informational and educational purposes only. It is not intended to be a replacement or substitute for professional medical treatment or advice relative to a specific medical question or condition.

We urge you to always seek the advice of your physician or medical professional with respect to your medical condition or questions and before starting a physical exercise or dieting program

To: *Joanna, Christopher and Anthony,*

I hope you will benefit from my insights and ruminations on staying healthy as you get older...

ACKNOWLEDGEMENTS

To supplement my own experience of nutrition, exercise and other health-related fields I enlisted the help of many people who generously gave their time. These included:

Danielle R. Bouchard, PhD, CEP, Faculty of Kinesiology, University of New Brunswick. Bonnie Fulton, Wellness Branch, Government of New Brunswick. Dr. Kevin Christie, MD. Richard Louis, MD, NB Trauma Program. Tony Tremblay, PhD, St. Thomas University. Dr Etienne Richer, McGill University.

A special acknowledgment goes to Deborah, my wife and companion for over 34 years. Without her help and commitment to health and nutrition - not to mention her wonderful cooking skills - I would not have written this book.

In addition to the subject matter experts I consulted, every health concept that I refer to in 'Forty plus Thirty' has been carefully researched. There is a list of key sources used in the 'References' section at the end of the book.

Forward

The goal of this book is to show how you can remain in good health and continue to enjoy life in spite of getting older. It's based on my own personal experience - I've maintained a high level of health and wellness to the age of 76 and hopefully well beyond.

I firmly believe that improving our health and fitness levels and increasing our lifespan is well within the grasp of most of us. Even if you are having some minor health problems today, you should still be able to look forward to reaching your later years full of vitality and enthusiasm for life.

Our perception of old age has radically changed over the years. Prior to modernization and the mass move to urban living, older people worked more, generally enjoyed good health and were more accepted by the rest of society. These days most of us associate old age with an inevitable decline of physical and mental abilities, leading to a very dependent lifestyle that relies on medical intervention, nursing homes and family support.

Although this perception itself may be correct, the above outcome is not a foregone conclusion. We <u>can</u> enjoy full and active lives well into our eighties providing we take better care of ourselves - starting right now, whatever our age.

I hope my story and the information I present in this book will serve as a lifestyle inspiration to everyone in their forties and beyond.

TABLE OF CONTENTS

Introduction

I am lucky. At age 76 I'm in good health, still fit and energetic and am not taking any medications. Now I certainly didn't plan this in advance. In fact when I was younger I didn't exercise enough, I drank too much and had a terrible diet compared to what I eat today. Fortunately I started to modify my lifestyle and gradually improve my health over the years. My goal in writing this book is to show you how I did this and what you can do to remain fit and healthy and enjoy life as you get older.

Please don't think this is just another 'diet and exercise ' book. Obviously both of these can play a huge role in our health and wellness and I talk about them a lot. But when it comes to Wellness there are other important factors that come into play - our mental outlook on life, our stress levels, our genes and much more. I'll be discussing each of these in detail as I go through the book.

Information Overload

How many self-help and fitness books are available today - thousands? The Internet is overloaded with websites telling us how to live right, how to lose weight, how to eat right... In fact for every human activity there's probably a website telling you how to do it properly. There's also plenty of iPhone apps helping us to achieve these same things.

So with all the information on health and wellness out there (compared to say, 50 years ago) why are we a lot less fit than our grandparents were?

Again there are numerous reasons, but one of them is certainly not the lack of information. Our sedentary lifestyle is a big factor in our declining health levels, but it's mainly the lack of motivation and prioritization of healthy activities in our daily lives that are responsible. If we're not actually ill, we're not going to spend much time on activities that would help us avoid sickness in the future. We're too busy just 'getting by' from week to week. Sure, we might go the gym, or go for a run at lunch time and this can certainly help. But is it enough?

I just look around me as people are headed to work and I see the answer to this question in their faces, in their posture and in their weight. The basic fact is, as a culture, we're not very healthy. When you fast forward to the older segment of our society you can see clearly how you're likely to end up.

Less Happy

Apart from being less healthy, as a society we're not as happy as we were previously. (Based on a paper compiled by Sherman, Lyubomirsky and Twenge from surveys of 1.3 million Americans ages 13 to 96 between 1972 and 2014).

Younger people may be happier than their previous generations, but adults over 30 are not. While there are several socio-economic reasons for this, I think our generally poor lifestyle also plays a big role. Stress levels are much higher, sickness like flu and other minor infections are more common. Just getting through a typical workday has become a chore for many of us. As we age it does not improve and seniors today are less content than before. Old age is just not something we look forward to with any anticipation.

Take Action Now

In spite of knowing how we are likely to end up in our later years most of us don't do much about it. If you really want to improve the present state of your health and fitness don't just read this book. Instead, read the book and start altering your lifestyle. In fact if you've been sitting down for the last thirty minutes or more, <u>why not stand up now, take a break and walk around for a few minutes</u>. There are so many health benefits associated with this simple routine.

Did you do it - did you actually stand up and take a break? Congratulations if you did - that was a test to see how motivated you might be to changing some of your habits! As you'll see in later chapters, the real secret to getting and staying healthier is <u>you</u> - it's not your favorite magazine or TV show, not your doctor, nor your gym instructor and so on. Yes - these professionals can help a lot, but ultimately your future wellness and longevity are in your hands. Get used to this concept – you and only you, are in charge.

Why I Wrote This Book

I woke up one morning in early January of the year I turned 75 and asked myself what could I do to celebrate reaching the three-quarter century mark, which to me seemed like a big deal. After a lot of thought and rejecting several different ideas, I decided to write a book about being active and enjoying life at my age. Then I thought of some of my friends, including several younger ones, who were starting to have health issues. After doing some research on sickness and aging I was shocked to discover the discouraging health statistics for people living in North America.

I began to wonder why I should be any healthier than the average person. It was only over the last thirty five years that I'd started to pay more attention to my lifestyle. Before that, I was just like many other people - eating poorly, not taking the time to exercise properly and worrying constantly about one thing or the other.

Reflecting on my own experiences, I thought that there may be several reasons why I was healthier than the average 75 year-old. It could be because of:

- Good genes
- Better diet
- Frequent exercise
- Just being plain lucky!

But then another thought struck me. <u>Maybe I'm simply normal for my age</u> and it's the modern style of living that is causing many people to age faster and get sicker much sooner than they should.

I'm convinced now that this is true. Much of what we hear and experience leads us to believe that even though we may live longer (thanks to modern medicine) we'll still become weak and frail and probably end our years in an assisted living community. But this may not necessarily be a foregone conclusion...

I decided to write my book based on the theme that we don't have to face rapidly declining wellness levels as we get older. If we can start to make changes now in the way we live then we'll be able to enjoy a longer and happier 'old' age. I hope I can convince you to change your beliefs about getting older. If you can do this earlier on in life, in your forties and fifties (or maybe even sooner), then you'll certainly reap the benefits later on. Think of it like saving for retirement, you'll be accumulating plenty of credits in your health bank.

I'm not saying you won't get sick, or you won't end up in a nursing home, this could well happen. But it should be much later on in life as we reach the natural end of our lives. The current belief is that our biological age is fixed somewhere between 100 and 125 years. The oldest verified age was that of Jeanne Calment of France who lived to reach 122 years old!

Realistically, I don't think any of us expect to be around that long, but living a full and active life into our nineties should be achievable for many of us. I firmly believe that this is possible - but only if we start following a healthier lifestyle than the one we have today.

My Background

Before we get started on the main topics, I want to describe my own background to show that I'm just an average person and if I can get this far - so can you.

I was brought up in the post-war years in a small city in Northern England. We weren't well off by any means, but like so many others at that time managed to get by on a single income. In those days there were no supermarkets and I remember accompanying my mother when she went shopping. We'd visit the butcher shop or fish store, the grocery store, the baker and so on. Our milk would be delivered fresh to the door every day. We'd also get farm produce from the local market.

Looking back I now realize that we consumed way more fresh food than processed. We'd have canned food like some vegetables and baked beans from time to time, but that would be all. It was only as I grew older and the food industry developed, that I switched my own eating habits over to processed food because it was so much easier when it came to meal preparation. I didn't know much back then about healthy living and like everyone else at that time, I just assumed that most of what I bought was 'healthy'.

As far as exercise went, I enjoyed sports at school and I also did a lot of mountain climbing in the beautiful Lake District in northwest England. However, when I started my university years in London, my fitness level plummeted and I spent more time drinking beer than working out! It was only during my vacation times that I'd get back to regular hiking.

Once I started working I was doing practically no exercise whatsoever. To make things worse, I started smoking! By the time I was in my mid-thirties I was pretty much out of shape and needing larger waist-size pants as time went by. I moved to North America to continue my work on a large computer project and ended up living in Montreal in Canada.

As I approached the age of forty, which in those days was considered 'middle age' I figured I should look after myself better than I'd been doing. I went to the doctor for a check-up and asked if he could test me for cancer. When he asked *'which kind?'* I gave up on that idea. I did however mange to quit smoking and also gave up drinking hard liquor (I really liked a good Scotch whisky and occasionally I may still have one!).

For exercise I started playing racquet sports - tennis, badminton and squash. One day, after a particularly hard squash game my friend turned to me and said "Mike - you're purple". Mmm, I thought - I need to improve my aerobic level so I'm not getting out of breath all the time. I bought a pair of sneakers and tried running. 'Tried' was the operative word because I couldn't run for more than a few minutes without having to stop for a break.

However, I persevered and after a period of several weeks of building up I managed to run six miles in one go! Gosh I thought, how on earth do people do this and then run twenty more miles to complete a full marathon (26.2 miles)? It was beyond my comprehension... However I enjoyed running and it became my favorite sport. I learned a lot in the succeeding years and even ended up running marathons myself. It was through running that I started to take an interest in nutrition and I was more careful about what I ate. Although I still ate too much red meat and fried foods by today's standards.

We next moved to Toronto, where my wife and I happened to live close to a health food store. We bought a juicing machine and started to add a lot more fruit and vegetables to our diet. We also read a lot of books on nutrition and the power of food. Over the next sixteen years or so, our diet evolved to where we're at today.

One problem we found was that nutritional studies and reports would often conflict with previous guidelines and it was very hard to know what foods were really good for you and which ones weren't so good. In fact it's still like this today. I hope that my book will shed some light into this problem and help you enjoy a healthy diet.

So that's a brief summary of how I got to be where I'm at today. It took me 30 years - hopefully you can get there sooner.

Section I - A Dismal Outlook

When we're teenagers - we'll live forever

This section discusses the current overall state of our health in North America. Our society ranks poorly among developed countries when it comes to life expectancy - a full five years less than in Japan for example.

The obvious question this raises is: 'why is this'? Is our medical system at fault, or are there other factors that account for our declining health and early signs of aging?

Your Golden Years Could Be Tarnished

I'd rather be poor and healthy than rich but sick.

When asked about their concerns over retirement people usually mention two things:

1. Not having enough money to live comfortably
2. Health issues (and how to pay for them)

The first one depends a lot on your present financial circumstances, your prospects and your expectations. The second one is much trickier - even people who are healthy in their forties and fifties can run into serious problems later on. Not only that, even if we have no debilitating illness now many people associate old age with weakness, decreased energy, lower mental acuity and memory loss. The image of a hunched-over old person shuffling along as if every step is painful is unfortunately our society's view of what we can expect as we get into our mid-seventies and beyond.

Thankfully - it does not have to be that way at all! If you take the right steps now you will be enjoying your older years as much if not more than you are today. But before we delve into the details, let's take a look at the state of health in North America and Western Europe 150 years ago.

Health In Previous Times

We usually associate life in the late 1800's and early 1900's with disease and short life spans. In fact a shocking 1 in 3 children died before reaching five years old, mainly from infectious diseases. Once people were past the childhood years their life expectancy was much better, often into the 60's and beyond. (U.S. Life Expectancy tables - table 11, https://www.cdc.gov/nchs/data/nvsr/nvsr54/nvsr54_14.pdf).
This was less true for people living in urban areas where sickness and disease were more common and where people often died before the age of 50.

But have we really improved a lot or have we just swapped one set of illnesses for another?

Pessimistic Statistics

Current U.S. and Canadian health statistics seem to contradict my earlier statements about our ability to enjoy our retirement years...

More than 70 million Americans over the age of 49 suffer from at least one of the following chronic conditions:

- Cardiovascular disease
- Arthritis
- Diabetes
- Cancer
- Lung disease

Actually, as of 2014 an unbelievable 60% of all adults in the U.S. suffer from at least one of the above problems! (From a Rand corporation report - http://www.fightchronicdisease.org/sites/default/files/TL22 1_final.pdf).

According to the Center for Disease control (CDC):

- Almost 25% of people aged 65 - 74 are rated in fair or poor health

- About 40% of people in this age group have high blood pressure

- Over 50% of the total population in North America regularly take prescription meds

- About 40% of people in the 65 - 74 age group are rated obese, but a whopping 63% of all Americans fall into the overweight or obese categories

Why is being overweight so bad?
It's often a pre-cursor to diabetes and cardiovascular issues. Carrying excess weight affects your quality of life in many

ways. Even something as simple as putting on your shoes can be a problem. Arthritic pain becomes more common and you can forget about walking up that steep hill!

Your ideal body weight is based on your body mass index or BMI. It is a measure of your body fat based on your height and weight. Below is a sample of a BMI table (You'll find a more complete table with more heights in Appendix I. Also included is a metric version in centimeters and kilograms).

To find your BMI value, simply look up your height in feet and inches in the left hand column and then read across until you find the column closest to your weight. Your BMI is at the top of that column

BMI >>	20	22	24	26	28	30	32	34	36	38	40	44	48	50
Height Ft. In.	-------				Body Weight In pounds				-------					
5' 2"	109	120	131	142	153	164	175	186	196	207	218	240	262	273
5' 3"	113	124	135	146	158	169	180	191	203	214	225	248	270	282
5' 4"	116	128	140	151	163	174	186	197	209	221	232	256	279	291
5' 5"	120	132	144	156	168	180	192	204	216	228	240	264	288	300
5' 6"	124	136	148	161	173	186	198	210	223	235	247	272	297	309
5' 7"	127	140	153	166	178	191	204	217	230	242	255	280	306	319
5' 8"	131	144	158	171	184	197	210	223	236	249	262	289	315	328
5' 9"	135	149	162	176	189	203	216	230	243	257	270	297	324	338
5' 10"	139	153	167	181	195	209	222	236	250	264	278	306	334	348
5' 11"	143	157	172	186	200	215	229	243	257	272	286	315	343	358
6' 0"	147	162	177	191	206	221	235	250	265	279	294	324	353	368
BMI >>	20	22	24	26	28	30	32	34	36	38	40	44	48	50

Here's what the BMI values mean:
1. 18.00 - 24.9   Normal
2. 25.00 - 29.9   Overweight
3. 30.00 - 39.9   Obese
4. Over 40.00   Severe obesity

A rising concern these days is the increased occurrence of obesity in children and young people.
Surprisingly the U.S. ranks very poorly when comparing the general health of its population with other developed countries. Studies conducted over recent years have consistently shown the U.S. ranks poorly (31st in 2016) for overall life expectancy among the developed countries. Canada is doing better in this regard and ranks 12th. If you live in the U.S. then you can expect to live to an average of 79 years - five years behind the leading nations like Japan and Switzerland. (Sources: World Health Organization, National Research Council and Institute of Medicine).

But longevity is only one part of the equation - what's the point of living longer if you're not able to fully enjoy those years?

When it comes to overall health and fitness for people over 50, the U.S. fares no better. We have some of the worst rates of heart disease, lung disease, obesity and diabetes when compared to other countries.

Why?

There are many reasons for the relatively poor health and lower life expectancy of Americans:

- Inadequate exercise
- Poor nutrition
- High stress levels
- Pesticide usage
- Expensive Medicare
- Gun violence
- Traffic related deaths
- Drug overdose (including prescription meds.)

The last three items on the above list do skew the life expectancy somewhat because people in these categories are often younger. But people as a whole either don't know or don't worry too much about their health in older years - until it's too late. I believe this is partly due to a belief that our governments, along with industry and science, will work together to come up with cures for every disease. And we'll all live happier (and longer) ever after!

Not to sound pessimistic, but here's a headline from over 12 years ago:

Injected Cells Cure Tumors in Mice
2006-05-09, Los Angeles Times

(http://articles.latimes.com/2006/may/09/science/sci-cancer9)
White blood cells from mice that are naturally immune to cancer cured tumors in other mice and provided them with lifelong immunity to the disease... Researchers hope that harnessing the biological process could lead to a new approach to treating cancer

Actually, cures for cancer have been making headlines since the 1940's. Cancer is a very complex disease and there are so many different health organizations involved it's difficult to really know where we stand today as far as finding a cure goes.

Science will keep you alive - it won't necessarily cure you!

Let's face it, the main person who can help you to stay in good health is you. Based on my own experience and observations that's exactly what I'll be discussing in the following chapters. But first let's take a quick look at what I mean by being fit and healthy.

Wellness

'Wellness' is a term that has recently become popular and we see it used all over the place. Even governments have created Wellness departments. But what does the word wellness mean, exactly?

The World Health Organization describes it as:

"...a state of complete physical, mental and social well-being and not merely the absence of disease or infirmity."

You can find many other similar definitions out there saying basically the same thing. The key point is that Wellness goes beyond being physically fit and healthy to include the mental, social and physical aspects of your life.

The degree of wellness you can achieve in your younger years will directly impact your well-being in later life.

The good news (I sincerely believe) is that it's never too late to start, even if you're already in your sixties and suffering from one or more of the chronic problems facing so many North Americans.

Likewise it's never too early either to start improving your wellness. In our thirties and forties we are quite often under a lot of work pressures and stress. This is where the decline in our wellness really begins. If you're in this category I urge you to start prioritizing the important things in your life, which should include taking the time to look after yourself.

My Main Keys To Wellness

There are generally accepted to be seven main components to Wellness:

1. *Social Wellness*
2. *Emotional Wellness*
3. *Spiritual Wellness*
4. *Environmental Wellness*
5. *Occupational & Financial Wellness*
6. *Intellectual Wellness*
7. *Physical Wellness*

I will concentrate on the physical and some of the mental aspects from the above list. This is not to say that the other components listed above are unimportant. I just want to focus on the main ones that I believe have a significant impact on our general health and well-being.

1. Nutrition
2. Physical health
3. Mental health

plus ... Your Genes

Improving your wellness is not as hard as you think and the more you work at it the easier it gets. When I started exercising I was more interested in simply getting fitter and reducing the size of my beer belly. Then as the years passed I began to pay more attention to my diet and overall wellness.

I've included a fourth factor, your genetic code. Although with the exception of some less common genetic-related diseases, the significance of your genes in determining your level of wellness in later life may not be as important as you might believe. I'll discuss more about this in the section on genetics.

For you to achieve the best state of wellness possible, all three supports in the above list have to be in place and working together. Just like a three-legged stool, if one of the legs is weak the stool will collapse if you place any weight on it.

1. Nutrition

Out of the key wellness supports, the food you eat on a regular basis, has the most impact on how healthy (or unhealthy) you will end up being as the years go by. I used to think exercise was the key, but now I'm sure it's the food we eat.

The focus of the next section on Nutrition is for you to determine whether:

- you are getting enough of the right foods on a daily basis

and

- you are avoiding foods that are highly detrimental to your health as time goes by.

2. Mental Health

Today the term 'Mental Health' goes way beyond the narrow (historic) definition meaning that a person was acting within the normal range of behavior acceptable to society as a whole. The World Health Organization defines mental health as:

"...a state of well-being in which every individual realizes his or her own potential, can cope with the normal stresses of life, can work productively and fruitfully and is able to make a contribution to her or his community"

Common mental health-related problems today include:

- Stress
- Depression
- Sleep problems
- Anxiety
- Dementia
- Eating Disorders
- Substance Abuse & Addiction
- Bipolar disorder
- Schizophrenia

That's quite a list, so you can see why the mental side of your health is extremely important in supporting your overall level of wellness.

3. Exercise

This is the third support of my Wellness platform. Once we leave school and college, many of us give up on exercising altogether. We all know the value of regular exercise and it's positive effect on our health, but how many people actually do it? In my case I did very little exercise for over a decade between my early twenties and thirties. Fortunately I did gradually get back into it (or I probably wouldn't have been writing this book today).

There are many misconceptions and different ideas about keeping fit and which kinds of exercise are the best. Typical questions people ask are:

- how much exercise time per week do I need?
- should I do high intensity or low intensity workouts?
- which is best - aerobic or anaerobic exercise?
- should I exercise if I have a health condition?
- is exercise bad for my joints?

One big problem with starting any exercise program after a long period of inactivity is knowing how to start and how much to do. In the chapter on Exercise I talk about how I got started and what I'd do differently if I were to do it again.

4. Genetics

I believe genetics is a starting point only and is not the influential factor affecting our wellness that many people believe. To put it bluntly the vast majority of us are not predestined to get sick - we just seem to end up that way. Genes definitely do play a role in our health and fitness - but to what extent? For example, there are lots of people who have the 'obesity genes' but they do not become overweight. Similarly, people who have the genes associated with Alzheimer's only have a slightly higher risk of contracting the disease than those who don't.

We know now that our genetic makeup is important; we just don't know exactly which genes or gene combinations are the biggest influencers. In the section "The Inside Story" I dig more deeply into this fascinating topic.

~~~~~~~~~~~~~~~~~~~~~

Is Our Medical System Failing Us?

At first glance, North America boasts one of the most advanced medical systems in the world, with un-paralleled surgical advances, organ transplants and synthetic limbs. The pharmaceutical industry is continually producing new treatments for a vast array of illnesses.

But, as I mentioned in the previous chapter, the U.S. and Canada performs very poorly when comparing the general health of the population to other developed countries.

Why is this?

There are two main reasons that I see:

1. Our generally unhealthy lifestyles

2. A medical system that doesn't deliver

Here are some of the problems with our health care system today

- Highest health care costs per capita than any other country in the world
- More focused on treatments and cures than prevention
- Expensive drugs
- Overworked doctors
- Treating everyone the same, it's only recently that 'personalized treatment' has become recognized
- Medical, medication and lab errors are more common than in most other countries
- Many Americans do not have a physician they consult regularly
- Physicians are not paid according to the quality of the care they deliver

- Our Health Care system is not convenient - we lag behind when it comes to accessing care out of normal business hours without visiting a hospital, where care is more expensive

Symptoms Not Causes - Treatments Not Cures

To me this is the area where our healthcare is falling short. Don't get me wrong - our medical system is better than ever before, but it's not always going in the right direction.

Are we treating only the symptoms of illness and not the root cause? For example, do blood pressure medications really help solve your problem, or do they just <u>control</u> the blood pressure to get it back within a normal range? Meanwhile your cardiovascular system may still be comprised. Similarly, many medications for arthritis, or fibromyalgia reduce the pain, but don't get to the real cause of the problem.

Having said that, medical treatments do allow many of us with chronic illnesses like diabetes to live and enjoy many more years of life than we would have had otherwise. You do have to wonder though, how much money and effort is going into research to actually cure the causes of illness as opposed to treatments only.

Many research projects, especially clinical trials, are funded by the large pharmaceutical companies, who obviously have a huge stake in the product being tested. So you have to take the results accordingly.

From the drug manufacturer's point of view:

> *The ideal cure is a pill you take every day for the rest of your life!*

Side Effects - The New Disease!

All medications have some adverse effect on your body, often because of the concentration of chemicals in the drug. My mother-in-law suffered from arthritis since her sixties and took daily meds to alleviate the symptoms. However, later on in her life she contracted liver problems caused from taking her arthritis medicine and this eventually led to an overall failing of her health.

Generally speaking, if you are taking any medication daily you will be risking some kind of side effect, from mild to serious and even death. Combinations of drugs, even including nutritional supplements, can aggravate the situation and greatly increase the risk of serious side effects.

♥ *Health Hint*
> Make sure to discuss the issue of possible side effects with your doctor. Consider the alternatives and make the best choice of medication for you.

You'll even find drugs available whose sole purpose is to reduce the side effects of another drug! What if we end up with yet more drugs to alleviate negative effects from the side effects drug - where will it stop?

You've probably gathered by now that I'm not a big fan of our pill-popping culture. Sure, it's easy, it works and you can often get away without making drastic changes to your diet and lifestyle. But in the long run and this is what this book is about - your advancing years, is it good for you?

There is however a newer method of treatment that could help us to better manage the drug side effects issues.

Personalized Healthcare
This relatively new approach recognizes that medical treatments do not work the same for everybody. Personalized care uses genomic factors and other biologic information to assess the risks of contracting certain diseases and chronic conditions in a patient. It also helps to predict how different people might respond to different treatments.

This form of treatment is gradually gathering momentum in the medical field, but I think it will take quite some time before it becomes standard practice. It will also have a huge impact on the way medications are prescribed, which could lead to some push-back from certain drug companies.

Prevention is Better Than Cure

There's an old saying "*an ounce of prevention is worth a pound of cure*" and this is certainly valid when it comes to our health. So if our medical system is only partially successful in helping to cure us, it becomes our own responsibility do something about it. Besides that, do you really want your future health to rely on companies who have increased prices by hundreds of percent on certain products without any concern over the patient's ability to pay?

Notwithstanding the recent advances in personalized medicine, my belief is that the best thing we can do is to try our best to avoid getting sick in the first place. Knowledge of our own genetic makeup may help in determining what we can do to try and prevent certain illnesses.

However the cause of a lot of our illnesses is not because we have so-called 'bad genes', it is self-inflicted through our choice of lifestyle! Obvious examples would be smoking and drinking to excess. Sports injuries are also a very common cause of physical issues. But does anyone get called to account when they become sick because they ate too many burgers and French fries? I don't think so...

Throughout this book I'll be describing what's worked for me over time and what I'm doing today to stay healthy. The next section on nutrition plays a big part in this and it can do the same for you. Avoiding poor food choices can make a huge difference to your health and is probably the most important factor when it comes to improving your wellness level.

For example, simply cutting back on sugar consumption is one of the best things you can do. When I worked in the midwest I used to see people at work having a super-size Coke or Pepsi and a sugar donut at break time! And I thought my coffee and muffin was maybe too much...

Stress is another aspect of our health that we need to manage. Many studies have shown that stress is actually the root cause of a lot of the chronic illnesses that people start to develop in their sixties. This is particularly dangerous because of the delayed reaction - you're stressed today and sick tomorrow, so to speak.

Anything you do today to reduce your stress level will pay big dividends later on in your life. The chapter ' Stress is killing you - literally' goes into this in detail and provides several methods you can employ to reduce the amount of stress in your life.

~~~~~~~~~~~~~~~~~~~

Section I Highlights & Summary

Here are the key points from the first section you can take away.

Basis of the Book

This book is based on my own life history and how I came to enjoy good health and vitality at the age of 75.

Holistic View

This is not just another 'diet and exercise ' book. I've tried to take a holistic view of wellness including our mental outlook on life, our stress levels, the effect of our genes and many more factors that affect our level of health and fitness.

Information Overload

With all the information on health and wellness available to us (compared to 50 years ago) why are we so much sicker than our grandparents were? Maybe it's simply a case of TMI - Too Much Information and the message gets ignored!

Pessimistic Statistics

The U.S. ranks 31st for overall life expectancy among developed countries. Average life expectancy is just over 79 years, compared to 84 in nations like Japan or Sweden. More than 70 million Americans over the age of 49, (4 out of 5) suffer from a chronic condition like diabetes or cardiovascular disease.

Wellness

The World Health Organization describes 'wellness' as:

"...a state of complete physical, mental and social well-being and not merely the absence of disease or infirmity."

The degree of wellness you can achieve in your younger years will directly impact your well-being in later life.

The Main Cornerstones of Your Wellness

- Nutritional health
- Physical health
- Mental health
- Your genetic code

Symptoms Not Causes - Treatments Not Cures

Many times, we are treating only the symptoms of illness and not the root causes.

Side Effects - The New Disease!

All medications have some adverse effect on your body and if you are taking any daily medication you will be risking some kind of side effect. Combinations of drugs, including nutritional supplements, can greatly increase the risk of serious side effects.

Personalized Healthcare

This new approach recognizes that medical treatments do not work the same for everybody. Personalized care uses genomic factors and other biologic information to assess the risks of contracting certain diseases and chronic conditions in a patient.

SECTION II - Nutrition

"Let food be thy medicine and medicine be thy food." -
Hippocrates

Here is my perspective on a topic that is constantly in front of us every day, to the point where it is suffering from 'over exposure'. Which may be why not many people really pay enough attention to it any more!

The Power of Food

After I began running regularly and started to feel much fitter, I said to myself this is great for my health and I won't have to worry about getting sick.

This assumption was completely wrong!

In fact I know now that what you eat every day has far more impact on your well-being than how much exercise you do.

It took me a long time to figure this out. I shudder today when I look back at my post-run meals after a Saturday morning club run of 7 or 8 miles. I'd have things like a fatty steak with eggs and French fries at the local tavern, washed down with a beer a two!

I began to take more of an interest in health foods after moving to Toronto. My wife and I purchased a juicing machine and would make some delicious drinks from a mix of fruit and vegetables. (More on the benefits of Juicing later on in this chapter). Now, over the last 20 years, we have become a lot more health conscious when it comes to what we eat.

New-trition!

Nutritional knowledge has leapt ahead over the last few years. More and more studies are showing the benefits of eating the right foods and the problems caused by consistently following a poor diet. The difficulty facing the average person is trying to understand it all, since there are so many conflicting theories about what to eat. For example there are strong proponents of the health benefits derived from a plant-based diet. At the other extreme are the Paleo diet followers who make very convincing arguments for eating lots of meat and vegetables, while reducing the intake of fruits and consuming few grain based foods.

So which is true? Personally I think there is some value in both approaches and it depends on your own body composition and your health and fitness goals.

Your Wellness Goals

In my case staying healthy and fit was my main goal. Some people might also be looking to lose weight and others to bulk up. Obviously this will mean consuming different types and quantities of food. So some typical objectives you might choose from could be:

- Decrease your chances of contracting serious problems like cancer or heart issues
- Lose weight
- Keeping fit enough to exercise regularly and eating the right foods to enhance your performance
- Correct a health issue you might be facing and reduce your reliance on medications
- All of the above

But can these really be achieved just by eating the proper foods? Yes, I firmly believe this to be true - all of the above can be achieved by consuming the right foods on a regular basis. But you need to look at the big picture. Many diets aim only at weight reduction and in the long term can even be harmful to your continued good health. The focus should simply be on quality nutrition. Following this principle can automatically help people achieve their optimum body weight and size.

Food as Medicine

My own experience has also convinced me of two things:

1. **Prevention is way better than cure**

2. **Proper diet is an effective medicine**

Now before you dismiss this claim as just another health-nut misconception, more and more scientific studies are confirming that many natural (as opposed to processed) foods have all kinds of positive benefits for our health. In spite of this, there are still many qualified medical professionals who dismiss the whole thing as 'quackery'. There may be some truth in what they're saying, but they are definitely throwing the baby out with the bathwater, so to speak.

I'm not saying you can cure everything with the right diet, there is a definite place for pharmaceuticals in our health care. But I don't believe medication should always be the first choice for resolving every health issue.

Where To Start?

As I mentioned, it took me many years to reach the point I'm at today, but hopefully by reading this you can start improving your nutritional intake right now - today! Some of the diets and health recommendations that caught my attention years ago were:

- The Atkins diet (yes I actually tried this, but not for long!)
- The Power of Juicing by Jay Kordich - he died recently at 93 years old after being diagnosed with bladder cancer at age 25 and told he didn't have long to live!
- The Zone Diet by Dr. Sears - this is a great regime you can follow all your life
- Alive Magazine (this is heavily sponsored by the nutritional supplements manufacturers)

I won't debate the pros and cons of these here, but what they helped do was to get me thinking seriously about what I was eating on a daily basis.

I urge you to do the same - look at your eating habits from breakfast (you do eat breakfast don't you?) to bed-time snack. As an example I was eating peanut butter every day, which although it's very nutritious, does have high fat content and other drawbacks. So now I vary it with other nut butters like almond butter, or not have any at all.

The problem we all face is knowing which foods are good for us and which are not. If this was a simple decision - good or not good - it would be much easier. Here are some of my concerns:

- We're all different, some foods that are normally good to eat can be less so or even harmful to some people
- We don't have enough time to devote to food selection and meal preparation
- The food industry messages can be misleading, to say the least (more on this in the 'Label Lore' chapter)
- Nutritionists have diverse opinions on the best 'diet'. As I said before, you have the plant-based diet proponents on one hand, the Paleo diet believers on the other and everything in between.
- Nutritional science is always evolving and conflicting study results are not uncommon

In the not-to-distant future we'll all be able to hook up to a computer and get a personalized analysis of our food intake requirements, as well as those foods we should avoid. As an extreme example, think of how allergies like peanuts or seafood can be critical for some people. There'll also be plenty of apps available telling us what foods are best for us.

I also think food labeling requirements will become more stringent and hopefully better enforced. For example the word 'organic' when applied to food, has a precise definition from the U.S. FDA. But now we need something similar for the overused and abused term 'natural'.

~~~~~~~~~~~~~~~~~~~~~~~

Is Our Food Supply Healthy?

Does a bear live in the desert? Is snow black? Of course our food supply is not (very) healthy. There are a number of reasons for this that I'll discuss later, but I believe the main one is very simple:

Food manufacturers put profit before health

Now before they all rush out and sue me, let me define what I mean by 'health' in the above sentence.

I'm referring to:

- healthy ingredients according to modern nutritional science
- healthy animals used to produce meat and related products
- fish from a natural environment and mercury free
- fruit and vegetables grown in a healthy environment

So what exactly is wrong with the food most of us pick up at our local supermarket? Here's a few concerns to start with...

- Cattle, pigs and chicken are often raised on factory farms where thousands of animals live in very unsanitary conditions and are confined to small areas.
- Farmed fish are fed a grain based diet enhanced with antibiotics - how far away from their natural food is that?
- Much of the wheat and corn in foods come from genetically modified (GMO) crops and are sprayed with pesticide. Now personally I'm not convinced that GMO foods are bad for you - but who knows?
- MSG is frequently used to enhance taste, in spite of the fact that some people may have adverse reactions to this flavor enhancer.
- Sugar is another common ingredient that is overused. Do you know the average American consumes 130 or

more pounds of refined sweeteners like sugar and corn syrup in one year (source: U.S. Department of Agriculture). That's almost three pounds per week!

- Sugar substitutes like High Fructose Corn syrup are as bad (or even worse) for you than sugar - but the food industry uses them all the time, they are cheaper than sugar!

- Processed meats like beef jerky, ham and bacon recently got a bad rap from the Heart & Stroke foundation for their link to heart disease.

Now in their defense the food industry goes to considerable lengths to make sure the foods they produce are free from contaminants like e-coli, salmonella and other bacteria that can cause food poisoning or worse. However, they also go to great lengths to improve their bottom line!

Ever since the food industry world-wide boomed after the second world war, every organization in our food supply chain from farming to supermarkets has striven to become more "efficient". A cynic might define efficiency as getting more from less and that is exactly what's occurring in the food industry. Let's take a closer look at the agriculture sector. The idea is to increase the yield per acre by producing bigger and better crops, such as corn, soy, wheat and so on. This is mostly achieved by genetically modifying the grain seed.

The giant Monsanto organization has dominated the global market for genetically engineered crops. Forty percent of the world's GMO crops are grown in the U.S., where Monsanto controls 80 percent of the GMO corn market and 93 percent of the GM soy market. Chances are the bread you ate for your morning toast was made from wheat that was grown from Monsanto seeds.

Note: Monsanto was recently acquired by Bayer of Germany and the Monsanto name will be dropped.

The processed food companies are no better. By 'processed' I'm referring to the food you buy that is pre-packaged. This includes foods like cereals, peanut butter, frozen meals, sauces and so on. Do you know that processed food makes up 60% or more of the average North American diet? Unfortunately the food companies start out with reasonably healthy ingredients which are then doctored up with sugar, fat and similar products to make them taste 'better'.

Now, I wonder if we are craving foods like this because we really want them, or because that's simply what we've become accustomed to? I say definitely the latter - I used to love sugar and sweet treats until my late thirties when I gradually reduced the amount I was eating. Now I don't even like anything too sweet and steer clear of many desserts and cookies that are over-sweetened. So our tastes can change!

But even when some food companies do try to take the high road and produce a healthier version of a product, quite often their competition steps in and offers the same old stuff in a new package to try and grab extra market share. The big loser is the consumer!

Even some of the so-called healthy foods are not that great - just take a look at the long list of ingredients on a box of popular 'nutrition' bars. Likewise, most granola products are absolutely loaded with added sugar.

So as a consumer, what's the answer? The next chapter describes foods that are good for you - ones I try to eat every week

~ ~

Food Types

Carbohydrates

Carbohydrates are an important part of our diet that provide us with the basic energy we need on a daily basis. So whenever I see 'low carb' diets being promoted I often wonder where people following these regimes are getting their energy.

Now as a long distance runner I know that the body can burn fat for energy. The Paleo diet proponents even go so far as to claim that fat and protein are better sources of energy. I disagree with this, especially if you do any kind of aerobic exercise regularly.

Carbohydrates are divided into two categories:

- Simple
- Complex

Your body digests each of these very differently.

Simple carbohydrates are made up of basic sugars that often have little real value for your body. The higher in sugar and lower in fiber, the worse the carbohydrate is for you. The exception is fruit and certain vegetables. Although the latter are simple carbohydrates they are very different from other foods in this category like candies or cookies. The plentiful fiber in fruits and vegetables changes the way that your body processes the sugars and slows down their digestion, making them act more like complex carbohydrates.

Complex carbohydrates, like whole grains and vegetables, take more time for the body to break down and use. The longer this process takes the better it is for your body and it avoids spikes in your blood sugar levels.

So make sure you get your carbohydrate intake from foods like:

- whole grains such as multi-grain bread or whole wheat flour products. I personally look for sprouted grain breads.
- fruits and vegetables
- beans (but not baked beans in molasses or pork!)

Fats

Just like protein and carbs, fats are a very necessary part of a healthy diet. But before you dive into a plate of deep fried chicken, be aware you should consume the right kind of fat. There are two types:

- Saturated
- Unsaturated

Although unsaturated fats are supposed to be better for you than saturated ones, it's a bit more complicated than that. First of all it's good to know something about all the different kinds of fat.

Fat Facts...

1. Saturated:

Saturated Fats

Solid at room temperature

Animal Based | Plant Based
Fatty beef, pork, lamb, dairy products | Coconut Oil, Palm Kernel Oil

Coconut oil is good for cooking at higher heats

Saturated fats have been consumed for years, both as food and as fat for cooking. It is generally recommended that we consume less amounts of this type of fat. However there is little experimental evidence connecting saturated fat to heart disease. In spite of this I do watch the amount I'm eating, and try to cut back as I think other food alternatives (like fish) are better for my health on a long term basis.

2. Unsaturated:

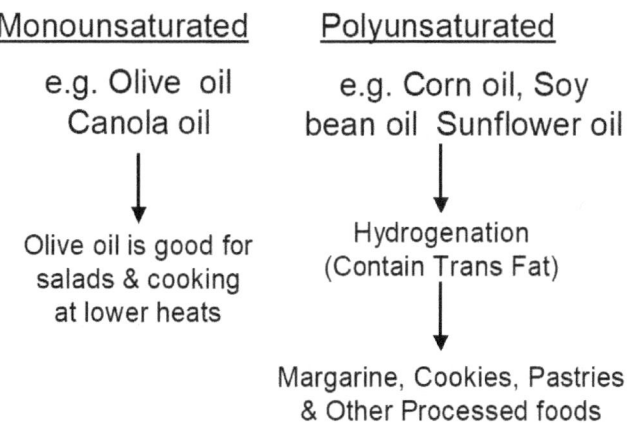

Unsaturated fats are generally better for you than saturated ones like animal fats. They help to lower cholesterol levels and tri-glyceride levels whereas over-consumption of animal based saturated fats have been linked to heart disease. You also need to steer clear of foods containing trans fats, most of which are artificially produced by hydrogenating vegetable oils.

Things get more complicated when we start using the different oils for cooking. Polyunsaturated oils are less stable and break down when heated, causing them to become oxidized and rancid. Saturated fats like butter are actually better for cooking, but should be used in moderation.

See Appendix D - Facts About Fats for a list of common oils and fats and their properties.

Essential Fatty Acids

We need to eat foods containing essential fatty acids – Omega 6 and Omega 3. These are commonly found in walnuts, eggs, salmon, vegetables, sunflower, corn, grains and meats. Healthy sources of these fats include:

- Cold water fish like salmon and sardines
- Eggs
- Hemp
- Flax
- Walnuts & Almonds
- Dark green leafy vegetables such as broccoli and spinach
- Virgin Olive oil, coconut and avocado oils
- Whole grain
- Lean meat

♥ *Health Hint*

> In North America, our consumption of Omega 6 fat compared to Omega 3 is way out of proportion. Instead of being the recommended 2:1 it is closer to 16:1 for the average person. So try to eat less Omega 6 sources such as dairy products, fast foods, processed foods, cookies, many cooking oils and red meats to name a few.

Butter from grass fed cows, coconut oil, lard, palm oil and olive oil are all relatively low in Omega-6. You can increase your intake of Omega 3 by eating more cold water fish and meat from grass fed animals only. Eggs from pastured chickens also contain more Omega 3.

~~~~~~~~~~~~~~~~~~~~~~

The Good

This chapter describes what I have discovered about foods that are definitely good for you, stuff you can eat frequently knowing that they are healthy, (but bear in mind everyone is different).

Superfoods

I hate that term! Maybe it's what super-heroes live on? To me it says eat tons of 'this' every day and you'll live forever. As far as I'm concerned most of the un-processed healthily produced foods could be considered a 'super food' because they're so hard to come by these days. The magazine 'Woman's Day' recently published a list of 52 superfoods, that's right 52! If you want to wade through their ad-laden web pages to find out what these foods are, here's the link:

http://www.womansday.com/food-recipes/food-drinks/tips/g2211/best-superfoods/?slide=1

For me, different foods have different qualities and health benefits. As long as you know which foods are healthy and which are not, you don't have to worry too much about missing out on any 'superfoods'.

Now that I've got that rant out of the way, let's get started on the 'good' foods!

Cold water fish like salmon, Atlantic mackerel, sardines and tuna.

These types of fish contain omega-3 fats, which are often deficient in the typical North American diet. Coldwater fish like this also contain vitamin D, which can be low in people living in most north American states and Canada.

Generally speaking, people who eat fish regularly are often healthier and live longer. The problem these days is that so much of the fish we buy comes from fish farms. I believe the quality is being compromised by all the grain and antibiotics they give to the fish. So avoid the 'farm raised' label whenever you can, you're much better off with 'wild caught' .

♥ *Health Hint*

What about mercury you might be thinking? Depending on the type of fish, the mercury level varies a lot. Fresh or frozen tuna is one of the worst offenders and you should only eat it about once a month. Here's a brief table based on data from the NRDC and the FDA showing how frequently you should eat different varieties of some common fish, starting with the worst offenders (most mercury).

Type of Fish	Consume...
Tuna, shark, swordfish, King mackerel	Eat less than once per month -these fish all have a relatively high level of mercury.
Canned tuna (Albacore), sea bass, grouper	Not more than three times per month
Canned tuna (light), halibut, lobster	Not more than six times per month
Catfish, flounder, haddock, cod, salmon, tilapia, trout, North Atlantic mackerel, shrimp, oysters, clams, scallops,	You can eat these often

Relative mercury levels in fish

(Here's a handy reference from the NRDC about mercury levels in fish https://www.nrdc.org/sites/default/files/walletcard.pdf)

On a side note, certain foods like cilantro and garlic are reported to be helpful in removing heavy metals including mercury from your body.

Eggs

In the past, eggs had a bad reputation because of the cholesterol in the yolks. At one point I would only eat one or two per week! The fact is eggs are a fantastic source of healthy nutrients. Ounce for ounce eggs are one of the most nutritious foods available. One egg contains:

- 6 grams of protein (compared to about 50+ grams in an 8 oz steak)
- 5 grams of fat
- Omega-3 fats (depending on the type of egg)
- 70 calories (compare to 50 - 100 calories in a slice of bread)
- Egg whites contain most of the amino acids you would find in red meat
- Anti-oxidants, plus vitamins A, B, D and E and minerals iron and zinc
- Phosphorous (which is good for your bones and teeth)
- ...and other important nutrients in smaller amounts

Never mind the egg - what about the chicken?
The downside (there's always a downside!) of eggs is actually the chicken that laid them. Birds confined to cages and force fed do not produce the same levels of omega-3 as chickens that are free to roam and fed a healthier diet. So look for eggs from organic free range chickens, or even better, a local farm that you know. They are well worth the extra cost.

Beans

Vegetarians have relied on beans for years to provide a nutritious source of protein, fiber and much more. But many of us eat relatively small amounts, in spite of recommended guidelines that say we should consume at least 3 cups per week. Over the last few years my wife and I have started to eat a lot more of this wholesome food. Thanks to her cooking skills I enjoy many very tasty bean-based meals!

By the way, if your workouts include running or other aerobic types of exercise did you know that beans are a great source of quality carbohydrates? So if you haven't tried bean dishes yet - what are you waiting for?

Veggies

As children we were told "*eat your veggies*" - for a very good reason. Vegetables are packed with nutrients like potassium, folic acid and many important vitamins. It took me a long time to realize this, but now I make sure I consume plenty of vegetables, both raw and cooked, every day (well most days anyway!)

Veggies of all kinds are incredibly good for you and for most of us we can eat as much as we want. But see my caveat on this further down. Here's just some of the benefits of consuming plenty of this nourishing food group.

- Can reduce the risk of suffering from stroke, cancer, heart disease and diabetes.
- The fiber we get from vegetables helps reduce blood cholesterol level
- Assists in the formation of red blood cells
- Helps maintain a healthy blood pressure

Here are just a few of my preferred vegetable superstars that we try to eat several times per week:

Spinach & Kale:

These dark green leafy foods can lower the risk of cancer, lower blood pressure, improve bone health and much more.

Broccoli:

A powerhouse of nutritional value - you can eat some every day!

Cauliflower:

Like broccoli it's full of vitamins and minerals. My wife sometimes uses mashed cauliflower as a substitute for potatoes! *Don't believe me? - Try it!*

Tomatoes:

Eat these both cooked and raw. Tomatoes are a good source of vitamins and minerals including potassium, magnesium phosphorous, manganese, and copper.
They have lots of health benefits, so eat plenty of them.

Avocadoes:

Avocadoes are really a fruit, but I've included them here because I relate them more to the veggie type of food. This extremely nutritious food is packed with many essential vitamins and heart-friendly monounsaturated fatty acids. Avocado is great when cubed and added to your favorite salad.

♥ *Health Hint*

Now here's a word of caution, although the above foods are extremely nutritious there are some cases where you should avoid eating them. For example:

- Spinach and cauliflower - if you suffer from gout avoid these and other cruciferous vegetables.

- Tomatoes - these are quite acidic, so if eaten in excess can lead to acid reflux.

- Avocado - some people can have an allergic reaction to this food

Fruit

Fruit of all kinds has many positive health benefits. Don't skimp on this important food group - I try to eat several portions per day. Here's a few of my favorites:

Strawberries
I usually have a couple at breakfast time. These berries provide a lot of health benefits and have been used for medicinal purposes since Roman times.

Blueberries
Well known for their anti-oxidant properties, they also help prevent the buildup of plaque in your arteries and improve cardiovascular health.

Raspberries
Like the other members of the berry family, this fruit has lots of nutrients and health benefits. We always purchase these when they're available.

Apples
An apple a day, as the old saying goes... My wife and I share an apple every day after lunch. Research studies suggest that apples could be one of the healthiest foods to include in your daily diet.

Bananas
Bananas are very nutritious and many contain essential nutrients like potassium, magnesium, copper, manganese and vitamins B6 & C. We usually share one at breakfast time

Kiwi
This tiny fruit makes up for it's size when it comes to nutritional benefits. Did you know it has twice the amount of vitamin C than an orange? It also contains vitamin E, seretonin, magnesium and potassium. Kiwi have become a regular addition on our shopping list.

Lemon

I've included lemon here because the juice has a lot of benefits. Besides containing many of the nutrients mentioned above it helps the digestive system and promotes smooth bowel functions. We include this every day in our morning drink.

♥ *Health Hint*

Try to eat organic fruit whenever you can. Especially strawberries and apples that are often heavily sprayed.

Teas

Teas are very beneficial to our health. I drink at least one cup of green tea every day. There is a lot of recent research showing that drinking tea regularly can actually improve your health.

Studies have shown teas can:

- Reduce the risk of heart disease
- Help protect against cancers
- Reduce the risk of developing Alzheimer's and Parkinson's diseases
- Reduce the risk of stroke
- Improve your cholesterol levels.
- and lots more...

Not bad for a little cup of tea, I'd say.

Some Popular Teas

Here are some of the more well known teas and the benefits associated with them. Contrary to what you might think, black, white and green teas all come from the same plant. It's just the way they are processed that makes the difference in the color.

Black Tea

Black tea has many healthy properties. It is full of micro-nutrients called polyphenols that can help fight against cancer cells and free radicals in your body. This tea is also credited with reducing plaque on your teeth and other bacteria in your mouth.

Green Tea

Green tea is full of nutrients and antioxidants that provide numerous health benefits. These include reduced cancer and heart disease risks, improved brain function and increased energy.

White Tea

This tea is credited with many of the same health benefits as the black and green varieties. It is thought to have more of the cancer-fighting micronutrients that green tea.

♥ *Health Hint*

All of the above teas contain caffeine, so you should bear this in mind if you are watching your caffeine consumption. Black tea has the most, with green next and white having the least amount. Compared to coffee however they contain much less caffeine. Black tea for example has about half the amount you'll find in a typical cup of coffee.

Chamomile

This herbal tea has been around for a long time and was enjoyed by the ancient Greeks and Romans. Chamomile is caffeine-free and has anti-inflammatory, anti-microbial and antioxidant properties. It is reputedly good for relieving stomach ache, helping with muscle cramps and promoting a good night's sleep. My wife and I usually have a chamomile tea every day as a bedtime drink.

Dandelion Tea

This tea is known for its help in treating a number of minor aliments such as upset stomach, joint pain, muscle aches and loss of appetite. It also serves as a natural laxative.

Rooibos Tea

This tea contains vitamin C and other minerals, as well as the polyphenols found in black tea. It is a good anti-oxidant and is claimed to fight disease and ward off signs of aging

♥ *Health Hint*

Many tea crops are heavily sprayed and contain pesticides. According to tests commissioned by the CBC (Canadian Broadcasting Corporation) program 'Marketplace' pesticide traces in some brands of tea exceeded allowable limits. See the full story here:

http://www.cbc.ca/news/canada/pesticide-traces-in-some-tea-exceed-allowable-limits-1.2564624

Try to get organic tea where possible.

Herbs & Spices

One of the arguments people make about healthy food is "*it doesn't taste as good as my regular food*". They're right - to a degree. Our taste buds have grown accustomed to foods that taste sweet or salty and usually contain a fair amount of fat. We find fried bacon and eggs to be very tasty, compared to say poached eggs. Having said that, if you are like me your tastes can and will change as you gravitate towards eating healthier meals

One way to counter the effect of switching to less fatty or salty foods is by adding herbs and spices to your meal. Many of the commonly used ones are also incredibly good for you. My wife uses them all the time. Here's a few examples:

Garlic

It might taste terrible if you bite into a clove, but it certainly adds a distinctive flavor to many prepared foods such as soups, roast meats and fish, stir-fries and salad dressing. We sometimes sprinkle minced garlic directly onto the salad.

Garlic has a whole lot of health benefits attributed to it, including

- **Anti-biotic** properties for killing bacteria and reducing infections
- **Heart-friendly** - by relaxing and dilating your arteries. It also reduces the formation of plaque in your blood vessels.
- **Cancer fighting** - helps prevent several types of cancer, like colon, breast and prostate cancers

Even if these are only partially true, it's worth eating frequently in spite of the odor on your breath!

Parsley

My wife adds this herb as a garnish to many dishes, including soups and salads. It is a good source of vitamins, including C, B, K and A. Parsley is good for your immune system and your bones

Basil

This is another of our favorite herbs and we often grow our own. It's distinctive sweet flavor is a great accompaniment to almost any dish. Like most herbs and spices, it's well known for its health benefits. It's a good source of essential nutrients including copper, calcium, iron, vitamins K and C and omega-3 fatty acids. It helps the digestive system and also has anti-bacterial properties.

Turmeric

This is the yellow spice you find in curries. It has been credited with all kinds of health benefits from treating

Alzheimer's to curing certain cancers. While these claims are scientifically unproven, turmeric does have anti-inflammatory properties that can help prevent disease. When it comes to cooking, you don't have to restrict its use to curries - add it to rice, soups, roasted vegetables and lots more.

Cinnamon

This is a popular spice often used in baking products like cinnamon buns and cookies. Like turmeric, cinnamon has powerful anti-inflammatory properties and it also contains large amounts of potent polyphenol antioxidants. This spice has also been credited with a wide range of health benefits, although studies have provided only inconclusive evidence of these effects. Personally I like the taste and when consumed in moderation I think it's good for you.

Black Pepper

Pepper is my go-to spice that I use all the time, instead of adding salt to my meal. I also use it often when I'm barbequing or making a marinade. Pepper has associated health qualities and may help prevent cancer. When combined with the spice turmeric this anti-cancer property is enhanced.

Chili and Cayenne Pepper

If you like a hot chili meal from time to time you're in luck! Hot spices have been linked to reduced risk of heart disease, slowing the growth of cancer cells and living a longer life! We often add hot sauce to our soup to 'spice' it up!

Ginger Root

This is commonly known for its use in Asian cooking, but we use it almost daily in a variety of meals like stir fries, baked salmon, juices and salads. Some people like to have it as tea by simply pouring hot water onto a slice or two of the root and adding lemon and honey if desired.

From a health perspective ginger is known for alleviating stomach related issues like nausea and diarrhea and for relieving pain from a variety of sources such as arthritis and chest pain. It's also good for the relief of sore muscles, if you overdid your workout for example.

While the above spices will definitely improve the flavor of your meals, do they actually have any real health benefits? The American Institute for Cancer Research has acknowledged the possible cancer-fighting benefits of pepper and other spices and encourages further studies in this area. I believe that in time, research will conclusively validate some of the health claims attributed to the regular consumption of spices.

~~~~~~~~~~~~~~~~~~~~~

The (Not-So) Bad

In this category I talk about foods that I eat from time to time because:

1. *They do have some good nutritional value*

2. *I like them!*

Beef

Like millions of north Americans, I love a good barbequed steak! But beef is one of the most controversial foods for a number of reasons. (Have you seen the Netflix show "Cowspiracy"?)

The main concern of red meat consumption is its reported link to heart disease and cancer. This is caused by high levels of saturated fat and carcinogens from cooking (especially on the BBQ). A recent scientific study showed the link between heart disease and red meat consumption for people with a specific type of DNA   On the other hand, meat contains many essential enzymes that we require to build and maintain strong healthy bodies.

I believe the real problem is not so much with the meat itself - it's the amount we consume. The average North American eats more than one and a half pounds of red meat per week. That would be like having three 8-oz steaks. I used to be in that category myself but started to cut back many years ago. Nowadays my wife and I usually share a single 10 - 12 ounce steak about once every week to 10 days.

♥ *Health Hint*
Look for grass fed beef, (or at the very least, beef raised without antibiotics and growth hormones). If you are barbequing the meat, always marinate it first - this reduces the amount of carcinogens.

Poultry

Turkey is a great source of lean protein. It contains all of the B vitamins, as well as potassium and selenium. Chicken is also a good source of protein. But both of these foods have a serious downside:

- The typical bird you purchase in the supermarket probably contains antibiotics and growth hormones. They are not always raised in a healthy environment. So try to find local farm-raised birds whenever you can.
- If you eat the skin (I know - it's the tastiest part!) be aware that you're consuming about six times more saturated fat than the lean meat.

Cheese and Other Dairy Products

I love cheese and eat some almost every day. However it is high in saturated animal fat and often contains a high sodium content. The good news is, dairy products like cheese, milk and yogurt are excellent sources of protein, as well as important nutrients like calcium, vitamin A, zinc and phosphorus.

If you can find dairy products from healthy grass-fed cows, so much the better. Try your farmers market for excellent locally produced cheeses.

Processed Foods - Part I

Technically, 'processed' food applies to any food that has been changed from its original, natural state in some way. By this definition pre-washed organic lettuce in a plastic container would count as 'processed'. Obviously the lettuce is a healthy choice and is good for you so I'm not talking about these kinds of products here.

Instead, I'm referring to a lot of the other foodstuff we consume on a daily basis, including much of what we purchase at the supermarket. The exceptions are the fresh produce, natural nuts, meats and fish. In fact someone said if we only bought the foods we found around the outside counters of the supermarket and not so much from the center aisles, we'd be a lot healthier!

But we all buy processed foods of one kind or another - they are so entrenched into our diet. They're convenient, always tasty and not always bad for you. You just have to watch out for too much added sugar, salt, fat and chemical additives and preservatives. When it comes to ingredients, I like to follow my totally unscientific principle - less is best! (Make sure you read the chapter 'Label Lore' for a heads-up on understanding ingredients).

Here are a few of the processed foods we purchase regularly:

- **Peanut and almond butter** - if you get the natural varieties the only ingredient they contain is the nuts.
- **Canned beans** like kidney, black beans and others. There's not too much difference between buying dry beans or canned and my wife buys both kinds. The dry ones just need more prep time.

  ♥ *Health Hint*
  > Canned foods may contain the chemical BPA which is linked to diabetes and other health issues. (See the Reference section for the Stamford University study or you can Google the article by searching 'Stanford study canned food')

- **Chocolate** - we love dark chocolate, anywhere between 72% and 90% cacao. Of course when it comes to chocolate it's easy to over-indulge!
- **Canned tuna and sardines.** We usually buy the ones packed in water. These fish both contain healthy Omega-3 fats, but we don't eat tuna more than two or three times a month because of the mercury content.

- **Canned tomatoes** - we use these a lot in cooking. My wife always looks for the low sodium ones.

- **Frozen Pizza** - you can't beat a pizza when you're pressed for time! We always buy the vegetarian thin crust variety like Dr Oetker's. My wife will often spruce it up by adding some other veggies like mushrooms or green peppers before cooking.

- **Chips** - yes, we love chips, but we try to restrict our total intake. A single 300 gram package will last us several days. I always look for those made with sea salt, a less processed alternative to regular table salt.

- **Crackers** - I go by the ingredient list and choose the simplest. Examples would be the Grissol brand, or rice flour gluten-free crackers, or plain whole wheat saltines with sea salt.

There's probably a lot more than I've listed here but the above are usually on our weekly shopping list. For the processed foods we never (or very rarely) purchase see 'Processed Foods - Part II' in the next chapter.

~~~~~~~~~~~~~~~~~~~~

The Ugly

I eat these types of foods rarely (or in some cases, not at all)

Bad Fats

As I said before, fat is part of a healthy diet. Unfortunately, most of the fatty acids we consume come from unhealthy sources, like saturated animal fats and common cooking oils containing hydrogenated fats. This can result in many health issues including heart diseases and diabetes. They also increase levels of the artery-clogging compounds - lipoprotein and triglycerides.

These bad fats are everywhere in our modern diet. Here are some common sources of these fats that you should avoid eating or minimize where possible:

- Hydrogenated oils found in fast food, margarine and other prepared food
- White bread and simple carbohydrates
- Trans fats caused by high heat when cooking with vegetable oils
- Deep fried foods (including your favorite French Fries!)
- Animal fat from eating too much red meat, pork, lamb and dark poultry meat

I haven't eliminated these completely from my diet, I still eat red meat and an occasional serving of French fries, but a lot less often than I used to. I definitely try to avoid hydrogenated oil and trans fats and most deep fried foods.

Processed Foods - Part II

This is a follow on from 'Processed Foods Part I' in the previous section. There are so many food products in this category that I'm only mentioning the main types.

Packaged donuts and similar pastries - usually contain a staggering amount of sugar and a high calorie count, 250 calories or more.

Many cookies and crackers. Cookies contain high amounts of added sugar, while many of the crackers have a lot of salt. They are often loaded with artificial flavoring, coloring and preservatives.

Processed meats. This long list includes things like bacon and ham (which my wife and I do eat from time to time), pepperoni and other dried sausage - they taste great but like all processed meats they contain nitrites which have been linked to certain cancers and heart disease. Personally I'm not sure that these meats are all that bad for you when eaten in moderation, but we certainly wouldn't eat them every day

Power Bars. These may not be as good for you as you think. I used to eat them all the time until I started reading the ingredients label. They often contain a lot of sugar and fat and although they are convenient I don't see them as a replacement for 'real' food. One bar I used to eat has about twenty ingredients, contains the cheap sweetener corn syrup and uses the questionable soy protein isolate.

Frozen Dinners These are often packed with added sugars, fat and sodium. The veggies look like they've been cooked until there are no nutrients left... Only eat these as a last resort!

There's a lot more I could add here, but you probably get the message by now - less is best! Always check the ingredient list and the amount of added salt and sugar when comparing different brands.

~~~~~~~~~~~~~~~~~~~~~~~

Label Lore - What's Really In Your Food?

It takes me twice as long to do my shopping nowadays compared to a few years ago. And no, it's not because I'm older and moving more slowly, it's because I've become a compulsive Label Reader. I read the label on everything I pick up before putting it in the shopping cart.

Why? Well it's mainly to check the list of ingredients, because I don't believe the food industry has my long-term health as its top priority. As I mentioned earlier, I'm a minimalist when it comes to ingredients especially the additives, even if they are apparently healthy.

A good example are added enzymes like protease which aids digestion of proteins. I've looked at products like crackers and one brand contains protease and the other doesn't. I don't know why this is so and I wouldn't necessarily choose one product over the other just because of this.

If you seldom read the labels on the foods you're buying, you might want to start looking more closely. Note that weights on the label are often expressed in grams (or milligrams for vitamins and minerals). There are just over 28 grams to an ounce. I use 30 for a rough estimate when I'm reading a label, so 15 grams would be about half an ounce.

Serving Size

Nutrition Facts
Serving Size 5oz. (140g)
Servings Per Container 2

Begin with checking the serving size on the label - the ingredient amounts are usually per serving. For example, if you have a can of soup and the label says it's 2 servings, that means that all the quantities shown on the label should be doubled if you plan on eating the whole can.

The serving size is very important when you are comparing similar products from different companies. You need to make sure you are looking at the ingredients information <u>for the same serving size,</u> otherwise you may be comparing the proverbial apples and oranges. It's also useful when comparing the prices on different brands of the same product.

Nutrition Facts

This section of the label tells you exactly how much of each of the principal nutrients you're getting in one serving. The label usually tells you how many grams of each nutrient are in the serving and what this represents as a percentage of the Food & Drug Administration's recommended daily intake (% DV).

Let's take a look at some of the key information on the label and what it means.

Amount Per Serving	% Daily value
Calories 60	
Fat 3.5g	5 %
Saturated 0.3g	2 %
Trans 0g	
Cholesterol 0mg	0 %
Sodium 160mg	7 %
Carbohydrate 12g	4 %
Fiber 0g	0 %
Sugars 2g	
Protein 1g	
Vitamin A 0%	Vitamin C 0%
Calcium 0%	Iron 4%

Calories

First off is the amount of calories, which shouldn't be too high. If you exercise a lot though, or do physical work, then you'll need more calories per day than the average person.

Fat

I always check this, especially when I'm comparing two or more similar products. It's best to keep the saturated fat in processed foods as low as possible. Stay away from food that contains trans fats as they are not good at all.

Sodium

AKA 'salt' - most of us get too much of this already, so it doesn't hurt to go for low sodium alternatives. Note that sea salt is reportedly better for you than regular salt, although there's no real evidence for this. However I usually pick the sea salt product if available.

Carbohydrates

This is a tricky one because it's subdivided into 'fiber' and 'sugars'. Now the recommended daily intake of carbs is 300 grams (roughly 10 ounces) - but the FDA was not thinking of added sugar when it came up with this number. Unfortunately the label does not distinguish between sugar added and sugar occurring naturally in the food. The maximum amount of added sugar you should be consuming is 25 grams per day for women and 37 grams per day for men. There's about 40g of sugar in a typical can of soda, so you can see that 25 - 37 grams of added sugar for the whole day is very little.

Protein

You won't often see a % DV for protein, unless the product is being sold as high protein, for example some power bars. Most of us get sufficient protein on a daily basis, but since I like to try and get some protein with each meal or snack, I usually glance at the number of grams of protein when I'm picking up a packaged item.

Vitamins & Minerals

Finally at the bottom of the label we come to the nutrients included in the food. I don't pay too much attention to this as I certainly don't know the daily values for each one. I prefer to get my vitamins and minerals from fresh products. However I do look at this section of the label just to get an idea of what is included.

Ingredients

Now we're getting to the good stuff! For me, this is the 'make-it or break-it' section of the label, where I'll decide to buy a product or not.

The ingredients are listed in order of their relative weight in the product. You'll be totally surprised when you check the ingredient list on some products - the main food item you're after may actually be in third or fourth place down the list.

Some ingredients you need to avoid include:

High fructose corn syrup (HFCS)

High fructose corn syrup is found in all kinds of processed food and drinks. It has been linked to obesity and cardiovascular disease and is worse for you than plain sugar. Even though some health experts say the evidence that HFCS is bad for you is not clear-cut it is still high up on my 'don't buy list'.

Corn Syrup and Sugar

Again, you'll find these in many processed foods. When it comes to your health added sugar is definitely your enemy. Over-consumption of sugar has been blamed for numerous health problems, including diabetes and heart disease. Choose foods with lower amounts if you must buy them.

Artificial Sweeteners

These sweeteners, like sucralose or aspartame, are all chemical-based and have no nutritional value. I always try to avoid foods that contain them. A Harvard Medical School article said "use of artificial sweeteners can make you shun healthy, filling, and highly nutritious foods"!

Monosodium glutamate (MSG)

Whether this is really bad for you or not is debatable and some people claim it's safer for you than salt. However it has been linked to health issues and allergies so I don't buy foods containing MSG.

Preservatives

There's so many out there I won't attempt to provide a comprehensive list. A rule of thumb I follow is that if the ingredient name looks like a chemical or you can't pronounce the word, then I probably shouldn't eat it. Ultimately it's your choice whether you do or not, but I've been cutting back on foods with preservatives. Here are some common ones you'll find in ingredient lists

- Benzoic acid
- Calcium Sorbate
- Erythorbic Acid
- Potassium Nitrate
- Sodium Benzoate
- Ascorbyl Palmitate
- Butylated Hydroxyanisole (BHA)
- Butylated Hydroxytoluene (BHT)

Artificial Coloring

Companies add coloring to foodstuffs just to make them more visually appealing. Look at all the orange cheese on the store shelves - the natural color of cheese is a pale yellow or white!

The dyes added to many processed foods are often made from artificial, or synthetic sources. Some of the more common ones such as

- Allura Red (Red No. 40),
- Tartrazine (Yellow No. 5)
- Sunset Yellow (Yellow No. 6)

reputedly contain carcinogens. Although the science behind these claims is not conclusive, I steer clear of products with artificial coloring just to be on the safe side.

Refined Oils

Oils from different sources are used everywhere in the preparation of snack foods, cookies, frozen foods and more. Normally these are supposed to be good for you since they are polyunsaturated fats, they are high in omega-6 fatty acids which can lead to increased risk of diabetes and heart disease when consumed in excess. The worst offenders in this regard are corn and safflower oil. But all oils have a drawback of one kind or another, so there's not much you can do about it if you eat processed foods. I avoid the corn and safflower oil and try not to overdo the snacks! For more information on cooking oils see Appendix D - Facts on Fats.

Conclusion

What I've learned from reading food label information is that there's a lot more additives in processed food than you might think - and many of them are synthetic. So when I compare one brand to another I usually opt for the one with fewer additives and avoid ones that contain any of my own 'don't buy' ingredients I mentioned above. Reward the companies who try to produce healthier foods by purchasing their products.

It's your choice though and it depends - how much do you want a certain food product versus what's actually in it?

~ ~ ~ ~ ~ ~ ~ ~ ~ ~ ~ ~ ~ ~ ~ ~ ~ ~ ~

Nutritional Supplements

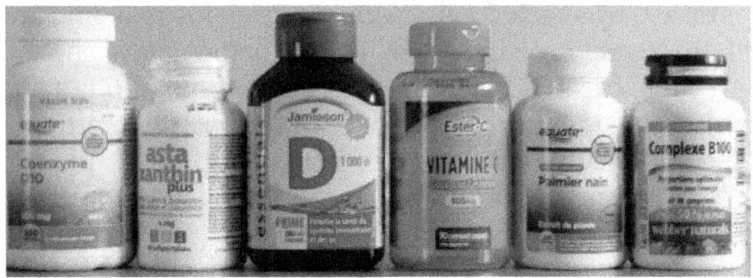

Should we be taking vitamins, mineral and herbal supplements? What a controversial question this has become! Before we get started on the topic, let me say that I have been taking supplements almost every day for 30 years and as far as I can tell it hasn't done me any harm. Of course if it hasn't helped my health in any way, then it's been a complete waste of money... Because I'm in good health at 76 I tend to believe that yes - taking certain supplements has helped.

But Should You Take Them?

The reason I started taking supplements in the first place is because I realized that my diet wasn't as healthy as it should have been. However although I'm eating much healthier foods than before I still take a few supplements on a daily basis. When you read the chapter on Essential Nutrients you'll see that for some of them it's hard to get the recommended minimum amount.

♥ Health Hint

> Some supplements can be harmful if taken in excess. They can also interfere with any prescription medications you might be taking. If you are taking meds <u>always check with your doctor and tell him which nutritional supplements you use.</u>

Here's a list of supplements that I take, or have taken in the past.

1. Fish Oil

Fish oil is an excellent source of essential Omega-3 fatty acids. Why do we need these? Because they play a vital role in regulating cholesterol triglyceride levels, in promoting heart health and many, many other benefits. The body has a limited ability to store these fatty acids and so we should consume them daily. It's also important to balance the ratio of omega-3 and omega-6 fatty acids in your food intake.

Here's what the U.S. National Library of Medicine and the National Institute of Health says about this:

> *"Western diets are deficient in omega-3 fatty acids and have excessive amounts of omega-6 fatty acids compared with the diet on which human beings evolved and their genetic patterns were established.*
> *Excessive amounts of omega-6 polyunsaturated fatty acids (PUFA) and a very high omega-6/omega-3 ratio, as is found in today's Western diets, promote the pathogenesis of many diseases, including cardiovascular disease, cancer and inflammatory and autoimmune diseases, whereas increased levels of omega-3 PUFA (a low omega-6/omega-3 ratio) exert suppressive effects"*

The ideal ratio of omega-6 to omega-3 is 3:1 or less. The average in our society is 16:1 and even higher in some people. The bottom line here is we need to consume more omega-3 fats and less omega-6. So unless you eat a lot of fish, this is a good supplement to take.

Check to make sure the fish oil supplement you choose also contains vitamin D, especially in winter time.

♥ Health Hints

1. The latest research is showing that taking fish oil in supplement form is not as beneficial as previously thought and can even be harmful if taken in excess.

2. Many of the fish oil capsules available are heavily processed and may not contain the health value they should. Also the source of the oil should not come from fish containing high mercury content. Read the label on this one!

Natural Sources
As always, if you can get your supplement naturally it's better than taking a pill. Here are some good sources of omega-3:

- Cold water fish like salmon, sardines, cod
- Flaxseed
- Walnuts
- Organic eggs
- Kale
- Brussels sprouts

2. CoQ10
Coenzyme Q10 (CoQ10) is an antioxidant that our body produces. However, as we age our CoQ10 levels decrease. Why do we need it? CoQ10 is used in the creation of an important compound called adenosine triphosphate (ATP) which is needed to maintain a healthy metabolism.

CoQ10 has been associated with a wide variety of health benefits - treating high blood pressure, reducing cholesterol levels and slowing down the progression of dementia and more.

However, except for helping in the reduction of high blood pressure, many of the benefits of taking CoQ10 have not been supported by scientific research.

Natural Sources
CoQ10 occurs naturally in these foods:

- Organ meats like liver, kidney and heart
- Beef

- Sardines and Mackerel (mackerel often has a high mercury content)
- Spinach
- Broccoli
- Cauliflower
- Peanuts and soybeans

3. Vitamin D

This vitamin is essential to the health of your immune system, nervous system muscles, bones and blood vessels. It may also help prevent certain cancers like colon and breast cancer.

The primary source of vitamin D is sunlight. People who live in northern climates do not get enough of this vitamin, especially during the Winter months. Fortunately you can also find vitamin D in fatty fish like salmon, tuna, mackerel, sardines and to a lesser extent in milk and eggs (See below).

The jury is still out on the benefits of vitamin D supplementation and too much vitamin D may actually be harmful. The recommended daily intake of vitamin D is about 600 IU's (International Units) or 15 micrograms. For people over 70 the recommended amount is 800 IU's.

There are currently large studies underway to determine whether this supplement can be helpful and in what quantities it should be taken. I rarely take this supplement any more, except sometimes in winter and rely mainly on sunlight and dietary sources.

Natural Sources

Only a few foods contain vitamin D naturally. Fatty fish like salmon, and tuna, or fish liver oils are among the best sources. Here are the amounts of vitamin D found in some common food sources

- Fish oil, 1 tablespoon 2000 IU's

- Salmon - 3 ounces 447 IU's
- Tuna canned 3 ounces 154 IU's
- Sardines canned 2 sardines 46 IU's

Milk and orange juice are often fortified with vitamin D as well.

4. Astaxanthin

Astaxanthin is a very powerful anti-oxidant that helps protect your brain and nervous system from free radicals and also promotes joint and skeletal health. Here are some of the other benefits attributed to Astaxanthin:

- Help relieve pain and muscle inflammation
- Supports eye health
- Promotes cell health
- Helps to fight tiredness
- Provides sun protection

♥ Health Hint

There have been reports of synthetic astaxanthin made from petrochemicals appearing on the market. Astaxanthin from this source is not approved for human consumption. The natural supplement is made from micro-algae, so make sure you purchase this product from a reputable retailer and check the sources used by the manufacturer.

Natural Sources

Astaxanthin is found in the following seafood:

- Pacific sockeye salmon - wild-caught
- Arctic shrimp
- Crab
- Crawfish
- Krill.

5. Glucosamine and Chondroitin

These supplements are marketed to promote joint health. As a regular runner, I started to take them as a preventative measure. However there have been no studies that suggest they actually work...

As a result I'll stop spending money on these, unless a conclusive study comes out that proves Glucosamine and Chondroitin do provide some useful benefits.

6. Saw Palmetto

The American Cancer Society states that prostate cancer affects about one man in nine. Some studies have suggested that taking the herbal supplement saw palmetto can prevent or reduce swelling of the prostate gland. Saw Palmetto is also beneficial for women - it may help block testosterone production, relieve menopausal symptoms and more. Like so many supplements however, there is no firm evidence that saw palmetto really works.

However in my case, I've been taking it for many years and so far my prostate is fine. I might be just one of the fortunate men who do not suffer from an enlarged prostate, but just to be sure I think I'll keep this on my supplements list.

7. Vitamin B Complex

This supplement contains all of the eight B vitamins:- B1, B2, B3, B5, B6, B7, B9 (Folic acid) and B12 There are many reported benefits from consuming these B vitamins:

- Promotes bone health
- Decreases stress levels
- Helps your brain to remain sharp
- Keeps you energized
- Helps prevent heart disease
- Is good for your eyesight
- Protects against allergies

♥ *Health Hint*

Drinking more than 1 or 2 alcoholic beverages per day decreases the level of B vitamins in your body. You want to make sure you are replacing them adequately through diet or with a supplement.

Natural Sources

The B vitamins are found in a wide variety of foods, so if you are eating a healthy diet, you probably don't need a supplement

- B1 - fruit, vegetables and grains
- B2 - grains, dairy products, fish
- B3 - potatoes, Portobello mushrooms, oatmeal and dairy products
- B5 - broccoli, turnip greens, tomatoes, yogurt, yeast, eggs, fish
- B6 - cereals, beans, poultry, fish and dark leafy greens
- B7 - fruit, vegetables, nuts, grains, liver, eggs and dairy products
- B9 - fruits and vegetables, whole grains, beans, breakfast cereals
- B12 - fish, poultry, meat, eggs and dairy products

8. Vitamin E

Vitamin E is an anti-oxidant and has several proven health benefits

- Helps strengthen your immune system
- Thins the blood and prevents blood platelets from clumping - reducing the risk of heart disease
- Fights fatigue
- Protects cells from damage

♥ *Health Hint*

Vitamin E is available naturally in many different foods (see below) so you may not need a supplement. In fact too much vitamin E through supplementation may be harmful.

Natural Sources

- Nuts and seeds - almonds, roasted sunflower seeds
- Green leafy vegetables like spinach and kale
- Avocado
- Wheat germ

8. Vitamin C

I've left this one to the last! I used to take a vitamin C supplement faithfully every day. Your body cannot store this vitamin and you need it on a daily basis. Vitamin C is needed for several essential functions in our bodies - growth and repair of tissues, collagen production, maintaining strong bones and absorbing iron to name a few. It's also an antioxidant, helping to protect cells from damage caused by free radicals.

Contrary to popular belief, fighting colds and flu' is not on the list of vitamin C benefits. There are no modern studies that support this theory. I was surprised to discover this because I always used to take a C supplement in flu season.

Natural Sources

Occurs in many foods including:

- citrus fruits
- kiwi
- berries
- broccoli
- tomatoes
- bell peppers

You can get the recommended daily value (DV) from just eating a single orange or kiwi fruit, or four ounces of broccoli. However the DV is only 90 milligrams which I find low, especially when the typical supplement contains 250 or 500 milligrams. Since I usually eat plenty of foods rich in vitamin C these days I don't always take this supplement.

Buyer Beware
So that's it for my own list of nutritional supplements. There are literally hundreds of them on the market today, covering all aspects of health and nutrition. This is a multi-billion dollar per year business, that is largely uncontrolled.

I'd been taking some supplements for such a long time I'd forgotten what the exact benefits of each one was! So if you are purchasing these products, take some time to research them. Even when I did that, I found hugely different opinions on the value of taking supplements, depending on whose website you're looking at. There's also large differences in the quality too - so always check the label for ingredients and source.

♥ *Health Hint*
> If you find a negative review of a supplement on a reputable pro-supplement site like Dr. Weil or Dr Mercola, then don't purchase it, unless your doctor prescribes it. As a case in point, I was researching the supplement Glucosamine - Chondroitin and found the traditional medical sites all said there was no evidence it worked. When Dr Mercola said the same thing - I was convinced. I figured if a guy who usually promotes supplements said it didn't work, then I wasn't going to buy it on the off chance he may be wrong!

Conclusion
So it's difficult to make a blanket statement about the value of taking supplements on a regular basis. I believe each

person's diet, state of health and physical exercise level can all come into play. Not to mention any genetic factors that may mean we need more of a vitamin or mineral than specified in the FDA's recommended daily value.

One thing I have learned is that the Internet can be a tremendous resource in helping you to decide whether to purchase a particular supplement or not. Just make sure you find websites that present different viewpoints. Popular pro-supplement websites include those from Dr. Mercola and Dr. Weil. I often check WebMd for a more traditional approach. If you really want an opposing perspective on this topic try Quackwatch!

Another good resource is your physician or other health professional with whom you consult regularly. They know a lot about your own situation and can match that to their knowledge of various supplements.

So, when it comes to supplements...

The truth is out there - it's just hard to find!

~~~~~~~~~~~~~~~~~~~~~~

Essential Nutrients - Where To Find Them

An essential nutrient is a nutrient that the body does not produce in sufficient amounts on its own and must come from our diet. Essential nutrients are necessary for our bodies to function properly. They include carbohydrates, protein, fat, vitamins, minerals and water.

Many of these essential nutrients are so necessary for our continued wellness that I decided to devote a brief chapter to a few of the more important ones. Some of them you probably don't know much about, or don't realize their importance to your health. Others we've discussed in the previous chapter on supplements.

I've included a table at the end of this chapter that shows the recommended daily intake of each nutrient and the best natural sources.

♥ Health Hint

Natural food sources are a much better way to get your daily intake of nutrients. Taking supplements for some of them, especially minerals, can lead to problems like toxicity. I never take mega doses (1000 milligrams or more) of any supplement. The only exception should be on a doctor's recommendation to treat a specific problem.

Magnesium

Not many people realize that the mineral magnesium is crucial to the proper functioning of our bodies. It is good for the heart, blood pressure, bone structure, preventing diabetes and it is needed in many key biological processes. In fact it is claimed by many doctors and researchers that magnesium is the single most important nutrient for our continued good health.

However, according to the National Institute for Health it's believed that over 50 percent (with some estimates as high as 80 percent) of North Americans are deficient in their levels of magnesium!

Some signs of low levels of magnesium in your body include cramps, weakness, headaches and poor appetite.

Zinc

This is another important mineral that we all need to stay healthy. It is present in every cell and helps your immune system to stay strong. It is needed for hormone production and digestion. Zinc is also an anti-inflammatory agent. Unlike magnesium however, many of us do get enough zinc from our diets. Some exceptions to this could be vegetarians, women who are breast feeding, older people and athletes.

Calcium

This essential nutrient is well known for building strong bones and teeth. But it also has several other important functions - cell division, nerve transmission and muscle contraction. We need a relatively large amount of calcium daily - 1000 milligrams. Dairy products are excellent sources of calcium and it is also found in lesser amounts in kale and broccoli.

Sodium

I've included sodium here because it is an essential nutrient. We need salt, a common source of sodium for a variety of vital functions in the body. Sodium is needed for muscles and nerves by facilitating muscular contraction and transmission of nerve signals. In the correct amount it is used to maintain proper blood pressure and helps to regulate the blood pH level. It is also used in regulating thyroid, pancreas and other gland activity.

The problem is we eat way too much salt, which then starts to have negative effects everywhere in your body where it's supposed to be needed. The maximum daily intake of sodium should not exceed 2,400 milligrams, (a serving of chips has about 160 milligrams). But there's salt in almost everything we eat so it soon adds up!

Common table salt and a lot of sodium in processed foods is also very refined, although it does have added iodine which is an important nutrient. Sea salt is a more natural source of sodium and contains important trace minerals like iron, iodine, manganese and zinc.

Potassium
Like the other minerals above, potassium is necessary for your cells, tissues and organs to work properly. It's good for your heart health, bone health, digestion and lots more.

Potassium is important because it helps regulate the sodium in your body. A proper ratio of sodium to potassium can help to prevent high blood pressure. In spite of it's presence in many common foods most people do not get enough potassium in relation to their salt intake.

Vitamin A
This vitamin is vital to our good health and longevity. It's needed in many different areas and functions of the body, including eye health, bone growth, healthy teeth, a strong immune system and much more. It's also necessary for fighting off infections. A deficiency of this nutrient in people in developed nations is rare.

Vitamin C
Vitamin C is used for tissue growth and repair in your body. It helps in the body's production of collagen, which is needed to make skin, cartilage, tendons, ligaments and blood vessels. Vitamin C is a powerful ant-oxidant and some studies have indicated that diets high in sources of this vitamin help fight cancer.

Contrary to a widely-held belief however, vitamin C will not help to prevent or cure the common cold. Nevertheless, it is an important nutrient that is widely available in many foods.

Vitamin E

This vitamin is another powerful anti-oxidant used to fight free radicals in the body. It is needed by our immune system and for maintaining healthy skin and good vision. It's claimed that vitamin E can also fight heart disease, Alzheimer's, prostate cancer, diabetes and other health issues. However there is no conclusive evidence to back up these claims.

Folic Acid (Vitamin B9)

Vitamin B9 has numerous health benefits. It is necessary for proper growth and development and for nerve and brain functioning. It can help prevent heart disease, stroke, cancer and birth defects in pregnancy. It also helps in improving our memory - something most of us can use!

Water

I've included water here because of it's vital role in our health and the fact that very few of us drink enough water every day. It is needed to maintain healthy cells and to prevent fatigue. It's necessary for proper kidney and bowel functioning and to promote a healthy looking skin.

Daily Values

The following table shows the recommended daily values for each of the above nutrients, along with their highest natural food sources.

See Appendix B for a detailed list of the main food sources, together with the percentage of the daily value, for each nutrient. The appendix also provides serving sizes to give a more practical idea of the quantities you need to eat.

Nutrient	DV[1]	Top Food Sources
Calcium	1000 mg - Women 1000 mg - Men	Yogurt, Cheese, Milk, Sardines, Salmon, Fortified Cereals
Folic Acid - vitamin B9	400 mcg - Women 400 mcg - Men	Beef Liver, Spinach, Black-eyed Peas, Fortified Cereals, Asparagus, Brussels Sprouts, Romaine Lettuce, Avocado, Spinach
Magnesium	320 mg - Women 420 mg - Men	Almonds, Spinach, Cashews, Peanuts, Black beans, Peanut butter, Whole Wheat Bread, Avocado
Potassium	4,700 mg - Women 4,700 mg - Men	Beet Greens, Avocado, Potatoes, Spinach, Yogurt, White Beans, Mushrooms, Banana
Sodium	Recommended Maximum Daily Intake 2,300 mg	Salt is in a lot of processed foods, but I prefer those containing sea salt
Vitamin A	700 mcg - Women 900 mcg - Men	Sweet Potatoes, Beef Liver, Spinach, Carrots, Cantaloupe, Pumpkin, Red Peppers, Broccoli
Vitamin C	90 mg - Women 75 mg - Men	Red Peppers, Kiwi, Oranges, Strawberries, Green Peppers, Broccoli, Grapefruit, Brussels Sprouts
Vitamin D	600 IU - Women 600 IU - Men	Fish Oil, Salmon, Tuna
Vitamin E	22 IU - Women 22 IU - Men	Wheat Germ, Sunflower Seeds, Almonds, Peanuts and Peanut Butter, Spinach, Hazelnuts

Nutrient	DV[1]	Top Food Sources
Water	8+ cups per day	Use filtered water where possible and try to drink the proverbial 8 cups or more per day. An alternate measure is half your weight expressed as ounces. So if you weighed 140 lbs. you'd need 70 ounces per day or almost 9 cups.
Zinc	8 mg - Women 11 mg - Men	Oysters (provide more than the Daily value), Beef, Pork, Crab, Lobster, Baked Beans, Chicken (dark meat), Yogurt, Cashews

[1]Abbreviations: mg = milligrams, mcg = micrograms, IU = international units

~ ~

Smoking, Drugs and Alcohol

I've included these popular vices together, although smoking and drugs hardly qualify as nutrition...

Smoking

There's so much proven evidence about the health consequences of smoking, it's hard to believe why anyone would still do it. Unfortunately I see so many young people smoking these days. Cigarette smoking negatively affects nearly every organ in the body, it can be the principal cause of many diseases and it reduces the lifespan of smokers.

If you are a regular smoker here are some of the major health risks you are taking:

- Increased risk of developing lung cancer by 25 times the risk for non-smokers
- Increased risk of coronary heart disease by 2 to 4 times
- The risk of a stroke goes up by 2 to 4 times
- The risk of developing diabetes is up to 40% higher for smokers than nonsmokers

The list goes on, but I'm sure you get the message...

There's no doubt about it though, smoking is extremely addictive and I completely understand why many people still smoke, regardless of the dangers. Now I smoked for almost twenty years, but was finally able to give it up. I tried several times to quit before I succeeded. Here's what worked for me:

- I reduced the number of cigarettes I smoked every day to 4 or 5. This took me a few weeks to achieve
- Then one day I just decided to quit altogether
- At the same time I gave up things I associated with smoking like drinking coffee, or a whisky after work.
- As a substitute for cigarettes I ate a lot of popcorn and peanuts for quite a while

Not very scientific, but it worked! Believe me I'm so glad I was able to quit and if you're a smoker, I urge you to try everything you can to lose the habit.

Drugs

Unfortunately the use of so-called 'recreational' drugs has been on the increase for decades. It's hard to imagine when you look at the negative impact drug use has on your wellness. You suffer both physically and mentally. Drugs have absolutely no place in your lifestyle if you are serious about improving your health and fitness.

Even 'soft' drugs like marijuana can have serious downsides (lung damage, memory loss and learning impairment) if used excessively. I used to smoke this when I was younger but smartened up and gradually quit the habit. The funny thing was, it was easier to give up than regular cigarettes - which shows the addictive power of nicotine.

There was a popular anti-drug ad that first came out many years ago, which showed a photo of two eggs in a frying pan with the caption "Your Brain on Drugs"! That just about sums it up for my thoughts on drug use.

Alcohol

A lot of recent research has suggested that one or two alcoholic drinks per day are actually good for you. (Just don't drink a week's supply in one evening :-)) It's claimed that moderate alcohol consumption has the following health benefits:

- Increases healthy cholesterol levels
- Promotes healthy blood flow
- Has an anti-inflammatory effect on cell tissues
- May reduce the risk of cardiovascular disease

Since I'm fond of the occasional beer or two, I'm glad to know about the above benefits. There's nothing more satisfying than a cold beer hitting the back of your throat on a hot day. Red wine is also reputed to be good for you in moderate amounts. However if I were a non-drinker I don't think I'd change my drinking habits for the sake of the above benefits!

When it comes to alcohol, the real problem is to control the amount we consume at any one time. After you had a couple it's easier to accept a third drink and so on. I've started buying non-alcoholic beer - it took me a while to find a brand a liked. But I'll often start out with one in the evening and then have a regular beer with my meal.

For at least one month every year my wife and I abstain from alcohol completely. I like to say it's to give the liver a chance to fight back! Seriously though, over-consumption of alcohol can lead to as many serious health problems as smoking. So try to cut back if you think you're drinking too much.

♥ *Health Hint*

Alcohol has been identified as a carcinogen by the International Agency for Research on Cancer (IARC). Worldwide, 3.6% of all cancer cases are attributed to the consumption of alcohol.

~~~~~~~~~~~~~~~~~~~~

Section II Highlights & Summary

The Importance Of Proper food

What you eat every day has far more impact on your well-being than how much exercise you do. More and more studies are showing the benefits of eating the right foods and the problems caused if you consistently follow a poor diet.

Food as Medicine

My own experience has also convinced me of two things:

1. *Prevention is way better than cure*

2. *Proper diet is the best medicine*

Many scientific studies are confirming that natural (as opposed to processed) foods have all kinds of positive benefits for our health.

The Food Supply

Our food supply is not healthy as it could be. Mainly because food manufacturers put profit before health. Much of what we eat comes from factory farms and in many cases is less nutritious than the locally grown produce you find at farmers markets.

Healthy Foods

The foods you can eat plenty of include cold water fish like salmon and sardines, eggs, beans, whole grains, fresh fruit and vegetables.

Omega-6 vs. Omega-3

In North America, our consumption of Omega 6 fat compared to Omega 3 is way out of proportion. Try to eat less Omega 6 sources such as dairy products and red meats and increase your consumption of cold water fish, eggs from pastured chickens, walnuts and flax seeds.

Red Meat Consumption

The danger of red meat consumption is its reported link to heart disease and cancer. This is caused by high levels of saturated fat and carcinogens from cooking (especially on the BBQ).

Look for grass fed beef, (or at the very least, beef raised without antibiotics and growth hormones). If you are barbequing the meat, always marinate it first - this reduces the formation of carcinogens during cooking.

Processed Foods

Try to minimize or eliminate the following processed foods from your diet.

- Donuts, pastries cookies and candy usually contain a staggering amount of sugar and a high calorie count. Crackers and chips are loaded with salt.
- Processed meats like bacon, pepperoni and other dried sausage contain nitrites which have been linked to certain cancers and heart disease.

Food Labels

It's important to read the food label on everything you buy. Compare brands and look for the lowest sugar and sodium content. Avoid ingredients like preservatives and artificial coloring where possible. Reward the companies who try to produce healthier foods by purchasing their products.

Oils and Fats

Oils from different sources are used everywhere in the preparation of snack foods, cookies, frozen foods and more. Avoid hydrogenated oils as they contain trans fats. Refined oils are high in omega-6 fatty acids - corn oil and safflower oil are the worst in this category.

Nutritional Supplements

I regularly take a few supplements. Some of my favorites include fish oil, CoQ10, Vitamin D, Astaxanthin, Saw Palmetto and Vitamin B Complex and Vitamin C. The sale of nutritional supplements is a multi-billion dollar per year business, that is largely uncontrolled, so do your research before purchasing!

Smoking

Cigarette smoking negatively affects nearly every organ in the body, can be the principal cause of many diseases and reduces the lifespan of smokers. If you are a regular smoker your risk of developing lung cancer is 25 times the risk for non-smokers. If you are a smoker I urge you to try everything you can to lose the habit.

SECTION III - Keeping Fit

"You're only as fit as your weakest part" - Dr. Braverman

This section discusses the popular topic - exercise. However like most things there are pros and cons and you can end up with injuries from doing too many strenuous workouts. I talk about exercise benefits in general based on my own experiences. You'll also find a simple test to help determine your own level of fitness.

Exercise is good for you!

Diet and exercise have long been the mantra of most wellness advocates. And why not - to a great degree it is quite true that if you watch what you eat and exercise regularly, you should remain in good health.

While I strongly believe this, the general population obviously doesn't, or at least they don't believe it enough and aren't motivated enough to actually follow it!

So why do any exercise at all?

The fact is our bodies are built for sustained activity, not for sitting around most of the day. By excluding regular exercise from your daily routine you are hastening the aging process, decreasing cardiovascular health and for many people, increasing body weight. Exercise has also been proven to reduce stress - a common contributor to many health problems.

But there's one very important benefit of exercising that you don't hear so much about:

> *Regular workouts are essential for maintaining your range of motion as you age.*

While writing this book, I met many older people and their main complaint was not about the meds they're taking, or the treatments they have to suffer through - it's their restricted movement. They can't get about like they used to, they have difficulty climbing steps, reaching for things in cupboards, or even holding a cup of tea. That's what forces them into assisted living homes, or requiring in-home help. It robs them of their independence.

If you're in your forties or fifties (or even sixties) you may have a hard time relating to this. After all you're still quite mobile (I hope). What most people don't realize is that the crippling effect you see in an 80 year old is the result of an insidious process that began 30 years before. Little by little, your ability to walk, reach and hold is gradually declining, unless you do something about it. If you don't want to end up like that (or at the very least, not as quickly) then get started on a workout program today - whatever your age.

How long does it take to get in shape?

If someone asks me this I usually say 'two weeks' to get started and then I explain that after this time they should already be noticing a small improvement in their fitness levels.

But the fact is, we're continually 'getting in shape' and the only difference is the level we reach at any given time. To use a well worn cliché -

Fitness is a journey not a destination.

As you get fitter, you'll be able to progressively do more. Sometimes though we reach a plateau and improvement seems to stop, or even reverse! When this happens it's good to back off a little - you're probably overdoing things.

Also let's qualify the timeframe expectation a little. If you are not in good health or not very active, then it's going to take you several months or even more to achieve a modest level of fitness.

Your age is also a factor; the younger you are when you start a regular exercise program the sooner you'll improve your fitness level. It's also important to realize that just because you start to exercise and do the right things, good health will <u>not</u> automatically result. Your chances of improved health through regular exercise will definitely increase, but there are other factors such as diet and hereditary traits, that can still affect you negatively.

How Much Exercise Do We Need?

The minimum recommended amount of exercise we need has changed over time. I remember when doing a workout three or four times per week was recommended. But now it's expressed as how many minutes of exercise are needed per week! You'll find 150 minutes, or 2.5 hours is often quoted as the minimum.

The amount you need depends on a number of factors:

- Your age
- Your sport
- Your fitness level
- Your fitness goal

I strongly doubt that the negative physical impact of sitting at a desk for 40 hours per week, plus 'couch time' in the evenings can be reversed by a mere two hours or so of moderate weekly exercise. Don't get me wrong, two hours is much better than not doing anything at all and if you're just starting a regular exercise program then it's enough.

But I feel we should be doing some kind of workout on most days. The key is to vary the type, the intensity and the length of the exercise. If we did hard workouts every day of the week most of us would quickly end up injured.

Here's some of the different workout activities I try to do every week, depending on the weather

- Running
- Walking/Hiking
- Cycling
- Swimming (occasionally)

Another thing you can do to extend your exercising time is to fit in more non-sitting time and try to be more active during the day. Here are a few ideas to get you going:

- Climb stairs at work
- Take a break from your desk every 30 minutes.
- Park further away from the store when you go to the mall
- Have a stand-up meeting at work
- Try working at a stand-up desk
- Walk or cycle to work

I'm sure you can come up with lots of other ideas to keep you more active. Try to cultivate a habit of simply moving around more each day. Our culture has become way too sedentary.

Make it a Priority

Unless you can make exercise a priority in your daily life it will get bumped every time there's a scheduling conflict, which can happen way too often. Think of exercise as food for your well-being - you need some every day! Once you are used to doing regular workouts, you'll really miss it whenever you are unable to, because of other priorities or if you are sick.

Taking up a regular sport that I could do on my own (running) was a true turning point in my life. It put me on the road to thinking seriously about my health.

How much is too much?

I recommend that you try to at least double the minimum recommendation for weekly exercise. This would work out to about 4-5 hours per week. Just do it carefully. The 'no pain-no gain' crowd often end up with more pain than gain. As someone remarked "only too much is enough" The same holds true for many recreational athletes who always want to push themselves beyond their capabilities. I used to be as guilty as the next person. As a result I have also suffered through most of the common runners' injuries over the years.

The key for exercising at all levels is:

Train - Don't Strain

The trick is to know your boundaries, which is where you train just hard enough to get the most benefit without crossing the line into the injury zone. Before we go further into the realm of fitness and exercise, a good place to start is to assess your own fitness level. The following chapter has a simple test you can do to find out where you are on the fitness scale.

~ ~ ~ ~ ~ ~ ~ ~ ~ ~ ~ ~ ~ ~ ~ ~ ~ ~ ~ ~

The Fitness Quiz

How fit are you?

Answer the questions below to find out your fitness level.

Note: - *this is just a quick and easy test I put together to give you an idea of where you're at on the fitness scale. For a complete assessment of your fitness level you need to visit a gym and take a supervised fitness test.*

Before answering the test questions below, check where you're at with the following measurements.

1. Average Weight Table:

Are you in the average range for your height and body frame?

Height	Women			Men		
	Small frame	Medium frame	Large frame	Small frame	Medium frame	Large frame
4' 10"	102-111	109-121	118-131			
4' 11"	103-113	111-123	120-134			
5' 0"	104-115	113-126	122-137			
5' 1"	106-118	115-129	125-140			
5' 2"	108-121	118-132	128-143	128-134	131-141	138-150
5' 3"	111-124	121-135	131-147	130-136	133-143	140-153
5' 4"	114-127	124-138	134-151	132-138	135-145	142-156
5' 5"	117-130	127-141	137-155	134-140	137-148	144-160
5' 6"	120-133	130-144	140-159	136-142	139-151	146-164
5' 7"	123-136	133-147	143-163	138-145	142-154	149-168
5' 8"	126-139	136-150	146-167	140-148	145-157	152-172
5' 9"	129-142	139-153	149-170	142-151	148-160	155-176
5' 10"	132-145	142-156	152-173	144-154	151-163	158-180
5' 11"	135-148	145-159	155-176	146-157	154-166	161-184
6' 0"	138-151	148-162	158-179	149-160	157-170	164-188
6' 1"				152-164	160-174	168-192
6' 2"				155-168	164-178	172-197

Height	Women			Men		
	Small frame	Medium frame	Large frame	Small frame	Medium frame	Large frame
6' 3"				158-172	167-182	176-202
6' 4"				162-176	171-187	181-207

2. Your Pulse Rate

A lower pulse rate usually indicates a more efficient heart function and better fitness. (Although it can be too low as well!).

Taking your Pulse:

1. Take your pulse on the inside of your wrist, just below the thumb.

2. Using the tips of your first two fingers press gently on the blood vessels on your wrist.

3. Count your pulse for 10 seconds and then multiply by 6 to find the number of beats per minute.

3. Recommended Blood Pressure:

Normal blood pressure is between **110/75** on the low end to **130/85** on the high side. However as we get older our blood pressure readings tend to increase. Here are some average readings:

Age	Blood Pressure
45-49	127/84
50-54	129/85
55-59	131/86
60+	134/87

Your blood pressure will also vary a lot during the day. I have a simple home blood pressure monitor and I find my blood pressure is lower in the morning and higher later on in the afternoon. You also need to take two or three readings at a time and take the average for a more accurate result.

Now jot down your score as you answer each question.

1. Can you climb a flight of stairs without feeling out of breath? Score 3 for yes and 1 for no.

2. Check the weight table above. Score 3 if you fall in the average range, else score 1.

3. Do you exercise regularly? Score 3 if you do any physical activity on four or more days per week, 2 for 2 - 3 days and if it's only 1 day or less, score 0.

4. Do you include both aerobic exercise like jogging and anaerobic exercise like strength training, in your weekly workouts? Score 3 for yes, 1 for no and 0 if you don't work out at all.

5. Do you spend more than 8 hours a day sitting down? Score 1 for yes and 3 for no.

6. Is your blood pressure in the recommended range as per the table above? Score 3 if yes, 1 for no.

7. Take your pulse rate (see below on how to take your pulse), if it's in the 50 to 60 range, score 3, if its between 60 and 80 score 2 and 1 if it's over 80.

What's your Score?

- If you scored **16 or over** you're probably quite fit and in good shape.

- In the **10 to 15 range** you're not a couch potato, but you should look at increasing your activity level.

- **Less than 10,** you definitely need to start on a fitness routine - but check with your doctor first!

~~~~~~~~~~~~~~~~~~~~~~~

Starting A Fitness Program

So how did you make out in the fitness quiz? I remember a time when I would have failed miserably, due to lack of exercise and sitting at a desk all day! Hopefully you will be motivated enough to make improving your fitness a priority.

Before we discuss the pros and cons of various exercise types, let's define what we mean by 'fitness'. This word conjures up different images for different people - to some it's being able to run a marathon, while to others just climbing a couple flights of stairs without wheezing and running out of breath would be enough.

The official definition from the U.S. Department of Health and Human Services defines physical fitness as:

"*A set of attributes that people have or achieve that relates to the ability to perform physical activity.*"

Quite a broad definition, don't you think? So I thought I'd expand on this a little - here are some of the key 'attributes' that I see:

- Cardiovascular Fitness
- Muscular Strength
- Endurance
- Flexibility
- Energy level

A person's energy level can vary a lot during the day and from day to day. The amount of sleep you get and the quality of your nutrition have a lot to do with varying energy levels.

Fitness Goals

Many diet and fitness products promote weight loss or anti-aging as the main goal. Your primary goal should be to be fitter not to look better or younger. As your fitness improves and your energy level increases you will end up <u>feeling and being younger</u>, not just looking younger.

Even the term 'looking younger' needs some examination. The popular image of people in their late seventies and eighties is of a heavily wrinkled, hunched-over person, shuffling along with restricted movements. Who wouldn't want to look younger in that case! Actually many North Americans are aging long before their time, as seen when compared to their counterparts in countries such as Sweden or Japan.

Endurance Sports

I started running originally to help improve my tennis game - a sport I took up in my late thirties. But even though I could handle a couple sets of tennis, I couldn't run one mile without getting out of breath and slowing down. It didn't take long though (about a week or two) for me to reach a basic level of cardio fitness that allowed me to run a mile or two. Over the following months I gradually extended my runs until I reached six miles or 10Km.

I finally abandoned tennis due to a rotator cuff problem and recreational running became my main exercise of choice. I did end up gradually increasing my training runs and have completed many marathons over the years.

♥ Health Hint

> Running and similar endurance sports such as cycling have been related to Atrial fibrillation (Afib for short). Several of my running friends have suffered from Afib, but why just them and not others is very difficult to know. I'm convinced that it's not so much the sport itself, but more the <u>intensity level</u>. If you are continually pushing yourself and over-exerting, you are stressing your heart to a point where it can become damaged.

As most athletes know, it's a fine line between performance improvement and injury.

So always exercise within your limits!

Surprisingly I've always run my best races with the best finish times when I've been able to do that.

Endurance sports also increase the amount of free radicals in your system, which can lead to other health issues. So-called free radicals are simple molecules with an un-paired electron, which in excess are very damaging to other cells in your body. So make sure you consume plenty of healthy foods containing anti-oxidants like blueberries, strawberries, nuts and green tea that combat free radicals.

Resistance Training

Resistance, or strength training has long been a popular workout activity. For many years it was primarily a men's sport for bodybuilding, but because of the associated health benefits, it is now a common form of exercise among people of both sexes and all ages.

Also known as anaerobic exercise, resistance training differs from endurance sports (called aerobic exercise) in that it builds muscle using bursts of strenuous activity. Technically, aerobic means "with oxygen," while anaerobic means "without oxygen." For example when you run at a moderate rate, the oxygen you get through breathing provides energy to the muscles to be able to sustain the activity. However if you suddenly sprint, then you cannot provide enough oxygen to maintain the increased level of effort and you quickly run out of breath and have to stop.

Anaerobic exercise provides several important health benefits.

- helps build lean muscle mass
- can help improve fitness and endurance
- burns fat quicker than aerobic exercise

You don't necessarily need to join a gym or buy a lot of equipment to do strength training. There are many excellent workouts that I've done in the past using my own body weight. Exercises like push-ups, knee squats and pull ups (although you need a horizontal bar for this one) are all good examples of body weight training.

Yoga

I've included yoga since it has four important benefits:

- It improves flexibility
- It strengthens key muscles
- It has a meditative side
- It has a calming effect and helps reduce stress

I took yoga classes many years ago and quite enjoyed them. You feel incredibly relaxed after the session is finished. In fact at the end of the class I was in, the instructor had everyone lie on their mats and relax and more that one person would fall asleep!

I do some yoga-based exercises in my morning stretches and workout session. (See appendix E)

Racquet sports

Although this chapter is about individual as opposed to team sports, I've included racquet sports. Even though you need a partner to play with it's still very much an individual effort - and it provides an excellent workout using several muscle sets in the body, as well as a good aerobic capability. I took up running as a way of keeping fit enough to play a hard game of tennis or squash.

~~~~~~~~~~~~~~~~~~~~~~

Choosing A Sport

"Just Do It" - I really like this old Nike slogan. To me it says it doesn't matter so much which sport you pick - just be active and do something.

Years ago I chose running as a recreational sport for several reasons,

- you can run anywhere
- you can run outdoors year-round
- you don't need much equipment beyond a good pair of running shoes
- it gives you some 'alone' time, when you run by yourself

My advice to everyone who is not already exercising regularly is to pick a sport you think you'll like and will enjoy doing. It shouldn't become a drudgery just because you feel you must work out frequently. In fact if it comes down to that, you'll almost certainly end up quitting.

I joined a local running club and enjoyed the fellowship and camaraderie, as well as the friendly rivalry. Running with others is a great way to keep motivated and interested in the sport.

You don't need to do just one sport either, in fact cross training is an excellent way of keeping in shape and reducing the risk of injuries. My son's favorite is off-road mountain biking, but he goes kayaking frequently and is an avid skier in Winter. (I tried to get him into running, but he wasn't too interested!).

Motivation

I'll mention this now but will discuss the importance of staying motivated and focused in more detail in the 'Mind Power' section.

When it comes to fitness and health, many people start out 'gung ho' (usually in January) and then gradually slacken off until they drop out altogether. They lose their motivation and keeping fit or losing weight becomes less of a priority than it was before.

Three things helped me stay motivated after I started running:

1) A desire to run faster times,
2) Being a running club member
3) The idea of one day running a marathon

After a while running became so ingrained in my life, that I really missed it whenever I was unable to run for one reason or another. In a way - I was addicted to running!

Exercise With Care

All sports have associated risks and it's only recently that new evidence has come to light about some of the issues. There is a downside to regular running (and other endurance sports). Studies have shown that a prolonged effort like marathon running can cause scarring of the heart tissues and other problems. If you do aerobic exercises like running or cycling that is something you should be aware of and you should try to avoid too many long hard workouts.

For this reason it's best to consider alternatives like interval training. High Intensity Interval Training (HIIT) has become very popular these days as a way to increase endurance and build strength. However HIIT is not without risk and it's easy to sustain an injury. This type of intense exercise is best undertaken with a qualified trainer.

A condition called rhabdomyolysis (rhab·do·my·ol·y·sis) can occur if you start any strenuous activity program without a gradual build-up. Rhabdomylosis causes muscle tissue to breakdown and the contents enter the bloodstream. This can end up causing serious damage to the liver. Trying to run a marathon without following a proper training program, or doing an intense FIT workout without previous muscle strengthening are examples of overdoing a workout.

Typical Recreational Sports:

Here are some of the more popular recreational sports that people enjoy doing, excluding team sports:

- Running
- Cycling
- Walking / Hiking
- Aerobics /Interval Training
- Triathlons
- Weight lifting
- Yoga
- Swimming
- Mountaineering
- Cross country & downhill skiing
- Golf
- Tennis
- Badminton
- Squash
- Pickle Ball

Obviously, each of the above examples needs a different level of effort and makes for a harder or easier workout. Quite often people will have several different activities that they do on a regular basis..

What Sport Would I Do Today?

If I were to do it all over again, I'd still pick running but I would expand my range of workouts to include other activities like yoga and resistance training. I'd also cut back on the number of marathons I've ran, reduce my training intensity somewhat and take more rest days.

~~~~~~~~~~~~~~~~~~~~~~~

Avoiding Injuries

Remember the Nike slogan I mentioned in the last chapter? Well here's a new version I came up with:

*Just Do It - But Just Don't **Over**-Do It!*

Now before you say this is simply an over-the-hill old guy talking, keep on reading...

Know your Limits

I mentioned earlier about exercising "within your limits". I want to explain in detail what I mean by this phrase and why it's such an important concept.

First of all, if you've been doing any regular exercise at all you know that every day is different. On any given day you might feel great, like you could run twice as far, or do your strength training routine all over again. But other times it's a real struggle, either right from the get-go, or part way through your routine.

There are many, many reasons why this happens, including over-training, stress, the time of day, the weather and so on. I won't go into them all here, but the important thing is for you to recognize that this happens often and when it does, you are much more injury-prone. At this point you need to pull back:

- consciously relax your body - neck, shoulders, arms, legs
- slow down the pace of what you're doing
- cut the routine short
- take a break (e.g. walk if you are running)
- drink fluid - water or an energy drink

The key here is to be pro-active and don't wait until you are forced to stop, like all those marathon runners you see walking at mile twenty or later. If you do put it off your risk of an injury greatly increases. You are pushing your body beyond its limits for that day.

Now if you're an Olympic athlete in competition of course you're not going to pull back, whatever you feel like, because your objective is to win. But even elite athletes know what they can and can't achieve on any given day.

Most of us should be more cautious. You need to understand your body and how to interpret every discomfort, ache or moment of fatigue as you're working out and then act accordingly. By easing off when necessary and pushing harder when you know you're in good form you'll end up being much fitter and stronger than you would be if you just try to work through the pain.

So "knowing your limits" does not mean you should never push yourself. Instead it means recognizing when it's OK to do this and when it's not. As I mentioned earlier, pro-athletes like elite marathon runners know when to drop out of a race or when to carry on. When you have mastered this technique you'll avoid a lot of downtime due to injuries.

Over the years I've become much more attuned to what my body is telling me than I used to be when I first began regular exercising. I ran a half-marathon recently and pulled back on my pace after two miles, not because I was in any pain, but just because I thought I was going too fast. However by the halfway point I knew I could go faster so I increased my pace and finished the race with a good time (for me).

Sports Can Be Dangerous!

All sports are prone to causing injury and very few athletes avoid problems at some point or other in their lives. Of course if you play football or any contact sport, your injury risk skyrockets.

For some of the popular individual sports, here's a list going from most injury-prone to least. The assumption here is that the comparison is based on the same individual characteristics. (i.e. same age group, same gender, same intensity level, etc.).

Risk Ranking	Sport	Notes
10	Triathlon	This three-sport event has the highest risk. Tri-athletes have a 90% chance of suffering an injury
9	Aerobics	This high impact workout has a fairly high injury risk at around 70%
8	Running	Running is notorious for causing all kinds of injuries from the foot to the lower back. Over-use is the most common cause.
7	Strength Training	Not as risky as it may appear, especially if you use resistance machines and build up gradually. Free weights require a little more caution.
6	Yoga	I was surprised to find that yoga was a major cause of injuries, but it's true. Approach with care!
5	HIIT Workouts	These demanding workouts are the cause of a rising number of related injuries. Don't be too 'macho' when you do your workouts.
4	Cycling	Cycling itself is a relatively safe non weight-bearing way to keep fit. The danger is mostly from traffic, or from rough trails, especially in cyclo-cross.

Risk Ranking	Sport	Notes
3	Kayaking	A great upper body workout that is relatively injury - free. Knowing how to swim helps and wearing a helmet in white-water conditions is essential.
2	Swimming	Like cycling, swimming is a great non-weight bearing sport that is relatively easy on the body. Shoulder and rotator cuff problems are the most common injuries.
1	Walking	If you stay away from traffic, walking is basically injury free, unless you are a race walker.

Note:

The above table is my own assessment based on a lot of internet research of each sport. Also it is not meant to be a comprehensive list of all the different recreational sports that people do.

Whatever sport you're doing it's always good to know what the common risks are so you can take proper preventative or corrective measures early on. I've known people who have ignored the warning signs and then got injured to the point they were out of the sport for months or even gave it up altogether. Make it your goal to stay as injury-free as possible.

~~~~~~~~~~~~~~~~~~~~

Section III Highlights & Summary

Why exercise?

Our bodies are built for sustained activity, not for sitting around most of the day. By excluding regular exercise from your daily routine you are hastening the aging process, decreasing cardiovascular health and, for many people, increasing body weight. Exercise has also been proven to reduce stress.

Flexibility

There's one very important benefit of exercising that you don't hear so much about - regular workouts are essential for maintaining your range of motion as you age.

How Much Exercise Do We Need?

You'll find 150 minutes, or 2.5 hours per week is often quoted as the minimum amount of exercise you need to be doing. I feel we should be doing some kind of workout on most days. The key is to vary the type, the intensity and the length of the exercise.

Make it a Priority

Unless you make exercise a priority in your daily life, it will get bumped every time there's a scheduling conflict, which can happen way too often. Think of exercise as food for your well-being - you need some every day!

Fitness Goal

Many diet and fitness products promote weight loss or anti-aging as the main goal. Your primary goal should be to be fitter not to just to look better. As your fitness improves and your energy level increases you will end up <u>feeling and being younger</u>, not just looking younger.

Which Sport is Best?
It doesn't really matter so much which sport you choose to do, just being active provides many benefits. Pick a recreational sport you think you'll like and will enjoy doing. Team sports can also provide great workouts and are good fun, but you'll probably need to supplement this kind of activity with some individual exercise time.

Mix it Up!
Both aerobic exercise like running and anaerobic workouts like strength training are important and beneficial. Try to include both types in your weekly program.

Exercise With Care
All sports have associated risks and recently new evidence has come to light about some of the issues. For example there is a downside to regular running and other endurance sports if you overdo it.

Know Your own Limits
How much you can do on any given day depends on many things. The key is to recognize when your body is not up for a hard workout and ease off before your risk of injury increases and you may end up having to give up the sport altogether.

SECTION IV - The Power Of The Mind

"What the mind believes the body can achieve" - Anon.

This section covers many topics related to the brain and how your mind has a strong influence on how your body performs.

Mind Power?

Many people groan when the topic of 'mind over matter' comes up - they're convinced it's all BS. If you're in this group, I urge you to please keep reading. There's a lot more to this subject than you might think...

For example,

- Do you believe a strongly motivated person is more likely to reach their goal than someone who is less motivated?

- Did you know that some people who have taken a placebo during clinical trials have actually been cured - they believed they were taking the real drug!

- It's a well known fact that stress is the root cause of many illnesses.

These are all examples of how our mind can have a great influence over our wellness. The fact is, mental fitness is just as important as physical fitness when it comes to your overall health and well being. As I mentioned in the introduction to this book, I've been fortunate and have had a reasonably good mental outlook on life ever since childhood. Have I had problems? Of course I have - who hasn't? During my life I've had periods where I've been depressed, withdrawn, over-stressed and unhappy. But I've been able to come back and I'm convinced we can all do this with the right attitude and beliefs.

In Western countries we place a huge emphasis on physical fitness and it's something every school child is brought up with. But are we taught much about the mind, mental fitness and our spiritual outlook? Very little, if any. By contrast, Eastern civilizations have always stressed the importance of the mental side of life and our inner connection to each other and the world.

Why is this so important to our wellness? In the following chapters I'll talk about what I have come to believe - that a healthy mind and attitude is just as important (if not more so) than the physical side. Of course the mind and body are both intricately connected and one can help the other. However, none of this matters if you can't easily change the way your brain is wired...

Neuroplasticity

The good news is that modern science has shown that your brain has the ability to modify itself. Previously, scientists commonly thought that the brain stopped developing in adolescence. They thought the connections that were formed between the brain cells were fixed and stayed that way as we aged. Now we know this is not the case. Neuroplasticity is the term used for the brain's ability to change - it can re-organize pathways and create new connections. So you can teach an old dog new tricks, so to speak.

Why is this so important? As you read further in this section you'll see that a lot of what you do every day is driven by your current mindset. If you can't change this you won't even get to first base when it comes to improving your health and longevity.

Note:
> Although the neoroplastic process has scientifically been proven, a lot of the claims surrounding it have not. I personally think the we can definitely modify our thinking to create 'healthy habits', but this is harder for some people to achieve than others.

~~~~~~~~~~~~~~~~~~~~~

Self-Motivation Is The Key

I learned from my marathon running days that without a sufficient level of motivation you wouldn't make it through the training program, let alone run the 26.2 mile race. In fact without enough motivation, you're not likely to achieve anything. Yet surprisingly I've met many people who seem to lack motivation and they go through life on auto-pilot without any real appreciation or enjoyment.

I am stressing this because you must motivate yourself to take action if you sincerely want to improve. It's like the audience who listens to a powerful motivational speaker like Tony Robbins and walks out of the theatre thinking 'Wow - what a great talk'. Then two weeks later they've completely forgotten about it and their lives continue...

Why is this important to you right now? Well I assume you're reading this book because you want to stay healthy and enjoy your later years, which will most likely require you to make some lifestyle changes - starting now! Unless you can keep motivated to do this it just won't happen. So let's talk a little about what I've learned about this elusive quality called motivation that some people seem to possess naturally.

What is Motivation, exactly?

A very simple definition from the Merriam Webster dictionary is:

> *"The condition of being eager to act or work"*

The key word here is "condition". It's really a state of mind that everyone can achieve if they try a little. The rewarding side about being motivated to do something is that after a relatively short time the 'something' becomes a habit and you don't consciously have to make yourself act.

As a project manager in my working life I constantly needed to try and keep my team members motivated and on track. I quickly learned that what worked well for one person had little or no impact on another. We're all different!

I believe the solution is for each individual to motivate him-or-herself, given the right environment with goals they can relate to and understand.
I would first of all look for <u>de-motivating</u> factors affecting the team, such as:

- computers not working as expected (not that unusual!)
- noisy work areas
- other team members not readily available
- etc. etc.

These act like barriers to motivation - they can be overcome, but it's much easier to simply fix them first.

So if you're having a hard time staying motivated, take a step back and ask yourself 'why?'. It could be that secretly, you don't believe in the goal or the benefits you expect to receive. Or it may be something simpler like not having enough time, or being discouraged by other people.

Make It A Priority
Going back to my marathon training days, in order to stick with the program I had to make the training a priority in my daily life. This meant doing things a little differently - getting up earlier in the morning, running in poor weather, adjusting my work schedule and so on. My family was a big help in all this and it certainly made things easier.

So if you need to start doing more exercise as part of your lifestyle change, make sure you can fit the time needed into your daily schedule. If you don't plan how you're going to do this it probably won't happen.

Motivational Triggers

Even after we get started on something new we often falter along the way. It's at times like this that many people lose their initial impetus and gradually fall back to their old patterns. To overcome this, I would often think about running a successful marathon in a good time and this would usually get me out of the door for my long training run. Whenever you see that you're not keeping up with your program, think back to the reasons you started and try to re-awaken those feelings of enthusiasm and excitement. I explain how to do this in the chapter 'Making Positive Changes Become Habits'.

Visualization

This is a technique used by many successful people including professional athletes. It's a simple but very effective way of maintaining a strong level of motivation and commitment. You simply imagine yourself actually achieving the goal you are seeking. For an athlete this might be crossing the finish line ahead of everyone else, or standing on the winner's podium.

In our case, the visual image in your mind could be anything you'd like to be doing in your later life. Going for a brisk walk with your family, getting a great check-up result from your doctor, celebrating your 85th birthday in style, etc. You get the idea - right? Try it out, it's fun and it works.

Positive Affirmations

Many motivational speakers have spoken highly of this technique, which involves writing down a list of things you intend to do to achieve your goal. You then refer to these regularly to keep them at the top of your mind. In theory this helps direct your every-day actions to make the affirmation happen. For example to achieve a healthy lifestyle we could have:

- I'll eat only organic foods where possible

- I will eat green vegetables every day
- I will do some yoga stretches every morning when I wake up
- I'll only eat processed foods occasionally

Now many psychologists will tell you that positive affirmations just don't work. My take on this is that anything that even gets you thinking in the right direction is better than nothing at all. I've tried positive affirmations myself but personally I prefer the Visualization technique. But you should give them both a try and see which one helps you the most.

~~~~~~~~~~~~~~~~~~~~~

Brain Health

Introduction

One of our biggest worries about getting older is a reduction of our mental capacity and in the worst case, getting dementia or Alzheimer's disease. As I got older, I often wondered if a decline in my brain's abilities would be inevitable. The good news is I believe now there's a lot we can do to slow down or maybe even prevent this from happening.

Your brain, just like your body, benefits from exercise. It's like that old saying 'use it or lose it'. Since our brain and body are intricately connected, exercising the body is good for the brain and doing mental exercises to improve brain health is also good for the body. Some of the important chemicals our brain produces are:

1. **Dopamine** - helps keep you motivated, focused and energetic
2. **Acetylcholine** - a deficiency of this important chemical can lead to liver and heart problems
3. **GABA** - essential for calming the nerves, reducing anxiety and helping us sleep better
4. **Seretonin** - adequate seretonin levels are needed to maintain a positive outlook and promote restful sleep

A deficiency in any of these can lead to physical illness and disease.

Mind Over Matter

Why is your brain health so important? Your brain is responsible for the production of many hormones and bio-chemicals that have a profound effect on the health and aging of your body. The faster your brain ages - the older you will look and feel. Your cognitive abilities will also start to be impaired.

However, I know from my own and many of my friends' experience, that exercise (in moderation) can help keep our brains and consequently our bodies remain young and active. The right diet can have an even greater impact.

I first came across the fascinating topic of the brain-body relationship and the importance of a healthy brain, in a book titled "Younger You" by Dr. Braverman. It's well worth a read even though it was first published in 2007. After reading it I was convinced that taking care of your brain health was just as important as going for regular workouts. Now Braverman does have some detractors, mainly due to the lack of studies to support some of his claims.

Brain Health

Getting back to the main topics of this chapter - ways to keep an active mind, improve your memory and stave off dementia, let's look in more detail at seven key things we can all do to help achieve this.

1. Regular Physical Exercise

Studies show that regular exercise and aerobic exercise especially, provides many health benefits for your brain. Here are some examples:

- Increased heart rate sends more blood to the brain
- Helps the body release hormones that positively affect the brain
- Promotes the growth of neural connections
- Reduces stress levels
- Helps improve memory and learning ability
- Reduces the amount of brain shrinkage as we age

In fact some experts claim that aerobic exercise actually strengthens and helps grow brain cells, including those associated with memory. I hope this convinces you to get out and do some exercise. Even 20 minutes a day helps.

2. Brain Exercises

The brain is a complex organ, divided into separate parts that handle different mental functions, including:

- Memory and recall
- Our ability to focus on a task
- Intelligence
- Spatial ability
- Social skills

Equally important for a healthy brain is brain speed - how fast your brain processes information.

There are many mental tests and games that can help you improve your brain's ability in each of the above areas. Here's a quick example that tests your brain speed and language ability.

The following table contains words split into two parts. The first part of each word in the left column must be matched to the second part in the right column to form the full word. For example:

HAND	HLESS
BREAT	SOME

Answers:
Handsome
Breathless

How quickly can you find the following six complete words in the following sample test? (cover up the answers as you work through it!)

PARE	CURE
END	LSIVE
EFFE	LORED
COMPU	CTIVE
OBS	NTING
IMP	URING

If you got them all in less than 60 seconds you're doing good!.

Many people do crossword puzzles, Sudoku or play games like scrabble to keep their minds in 'active' mode. But don't wait until you are older to do this - your brain will benefit at any age. The key is to get your brain to try different things from its normal everyday thought processes.

Puzzle answers:
> PARENTING
> ENDURING
> EFFECTIVE
> COMPULSIVE
> OBSCURE
> IMPLORED

3. Eat the right food

It should come as no surprise that nutrition plays a highly important role in keeping your brain healthy. Here's a few tips:

- **Eat less sugary foods** (except natural fruit) - added sugar is bad for you generally and has a negative effect on brain function. It can also contribute to brain shrinkage.

- **Get enough omega-3 fatty acids** from healthy sources like cold water fish and organic eggs

- **Blueberries** are powerful anti-oxidants to help protect the brain against memory loss and decreased motor coordination associated with aging

- **Nuts and seeds** are another great brain-boosting food source. A recent Harvard study of more than 100,000 people showed that regular consumption of nuts (especially walnuts, almonds, peanuts and hazel nuts) was strongly related to longevity. Pumpkin seeds are also great to eat - they contain omega-3 and magnesium which has a calming effect on the brain

- **Vegetables** like spinach, romaine lettuce and cruciferous vegetables such as broccoli and cauliflower all contribute to slowing down the rate of aging in your brain. Other veggies like beets are also recommended

4. Reduce Stress
Prolonged stress is bad for your brain (see more in the chapter on Stress). It can lead to decreased brain volume and may increase the chance of developing Alzheimer's disease.

5. Check your blood pressure
Studies show that high blood pressure increases the risk of memory loss, decreased brain speed, dementia and even Alzheimer's disease. Both the systolic and diastolic blood pressure reading have an impact.
Now blood pressure varies with age so you should know the acceptable range for you, (see the blood pressure table in the Fitness Quiz chapter) and try to stay within the recommended limits.

6. Avoid tobacco, reduce alcohol
Smoking has so many well-known adverse effects on your health, that no-one today should be using tobacco products.

A recent study found that people who smoke have a thinner cortex than people who don't. The cortex is the outer layer of the brain and is responsible for memory and language. It's also the most highly developed part of the brain. The good news for people who quit smoking is that the cortex is able to recover and regain some of its original thickness.

Like tobacco, too much alcohol has long-term damaging effects on the brain. Continual heavy drinking attacks the brain's gray matter and affects your memory, which reduces your ability to plan and prioritize. The general recommendation is to keep your alcoholic drinks to two or less per day.

7. Be Social!

Many studies have shown that social interaction and personal relationships contribute greatly to maintaining a sharp mind, all through our lives. So to help your brain stay active, join a group, visit family and friends more often and participate in social events.

Like many of these kinds of recommendations there are no guarantees and they may help some people more than others. But my take on this is that since they are all healthy suggestions, it certainly won't hurt to include them as part of your lifestyle.

The following sections discuss brain age and brain speed and how you can assess your own abilities.

Brain Age

Brain age refers to our responses to various tests designed to compare the age of our brain to our actual age. The gaming company Nintendo invented a video game to measure your brain's 'age'. However the company does not claim that the game has been scientifically validated.

There are many tests available that you can try out. A good one that I like was developed by Dr. Vincent Fortanasce. His popular book "The Anti-Alzheimer's Prescription" describes how to prevent or delay this deadly disease.

Dr. Fortanasce's Test is reproduced with permission below. (See his website at http://www.healthybrainmd.com/)

The following test asks you 25 questions and based on your responses, evaluates your brain age and risk of developing Alzheimer's. Mark your response True or False to each of the questions below.

True or False

1. I get 7 to 8 hours (or more) of sleep each night.

2. I eat at least 5 or more servings of fruits and vegetables that are high in antioxidants daily.

3. I eat at least one serving of berries like blueberries, raspberries, or blackberries daily.

4. I eat baked or broiled fish high in omega-3 fatty acids (especially eicosapentaenoic acid and docosahexaenoic acid) at least three times a week.

5. I take fish oil supplements high in omega-3 fatty acids or flaxseed supplements at least 5 times per week.

6. I take folic acid supplementation with my daily multivitamin.

7. I take a low-dose of aspirin daily.

8. I drink red wine or grape juice at least 5 times a week.

9. I exercise most days of the week for at least 30 minutes each time (total of three hours or more of strenuous exercise weekly).

10. I read challenging books, do crossword puzzles or Sudoku, or engage in activities that require active

learning, memorization, computation, analysis and problem solving at least five times a week.

11. My total cholesterol is less than 200 mg/dL (5.2 mmol/L in Canada).

12. My LDL ("bad") cholesterol is less than 110 mg/dL (2.6 mmol/L in Canada).

13. I have "longevity genes" in my family, with members who lived to 80 and older without memory loss.

14. I am not obese (less than 20 pounds overweight for a woman; less than 30 pounds overweight for a man).

15. I eat a Mediterranean style diet (high in fruits, vegetables, whole grains, beans, nuts & seeds and olive oil as the source of fat; little red meat).

16. I use olive oil and no trans-fat spreads instead of butter or margarine.

17. I have never smoked cigarettes.

18. I do not have diabetes.

19. I do not have metabolic syndrome (high triglycerides, central obesity and hypertension), also called insulin resistance syndrome.

20. I do not have a sleep disorder such as snoring or obstructive sleep apnea or untreated insomnia.

21. Daily uncontrolled stress is not a problem for me.

22. I have a strong support group and enjoy many activities with friends, colleagues and family members.

23. I have no problems with short- or long-term memory.

24. I'm ready to prevent Alzheimer's and am willing to do whatever it takes.

Now please go back and count how many of the 24 statements you marked "True." Here, we're aiming for a relatively simple means of tallying a score that will be easy to understand and apply to your diet and lifestyle habits.

Assessment

If you scored...

22 – 24 Congratulations! You are aging well. Subtract 15 years from your chronological age to find out your Real Brain Age.

You are presently healthy with a youthful, productive mind. Unless things change in your life, your risk of Alzheimer's disease is extremely low.

20 – 21 Not bad! Subtract 10 years from your chronological age for your Real Brain Age.

You are doing a lot to take care of your physical and mental health. Check the specific questions that you marked False – and be sure to pay attention to changes you need to make.

15-19 OK. Your Real Brain Age is the same as your chronological age. That said, you have a mild risk of Alzheimer's disease, so pay attention.

12 – 14. You have a moderate risk of Alzheimer's Disease. Add 5 years to your chronological age for your Real Brain Age. While there's not a lot of disparity between your Real Brain Age and your chronological age, you need to really understand the risks you have that increase the chances of Alzheimer's. It's important that you review the quiz and circle any of the statements that indicate some work is needed. Talk to your doctor about your risk factors you have, to see if treatment is indicated.

0 – 11. You have a high risk of Alzheimer's disease. Add 10 years to your chronological age for your Real Brain Age. Right now, call your doctor and talk openly about health problems you have. Ask if you're doing all you can to manage these problems. In addition, read the book 'The Anti-Alzheimer's Prescription" and flag those pages that may help to decrease your risk of Alzheimer's disease.

~~~~~~~~~~~~~~

Note: I'm not sure that questions 5, 6, 7, 8 or 16 are that critical since other healthy alternatives are available. However I reproduced the full test as is.

Brain Speed

Brain speed refers to the speed at which your brain processes and reacts to sensory information around you. Examples of this would be how well you remember a very recent event, or how quickly you react to dangers or answer a question. It's a proven fact that your brain speed slows down as you age, but regularly engaging your brain in different activities like mental tests will reduce the rate of decline. There are lots of these tests you can find online, but here's one you can do right now.

All the questions in this test contain a word and a picture. If these represent exactly the same thing check the 'Correct' box, if they're different check the 'Incorrect, one.

Now here's the tricky part, if the word 'Opposite' appears with the image you must do the opposite and check the box that represents the 'wrong' answer.

Here's an example:

DOG	Opposite	Correct....[ ] Incorrect [*]

Since both the word and the image match exactly - a dog, the right answer should be 'Correct', but because the word 'Opposite' appears then your answer would be 'Incorrect'.

This one is harder..

CAR	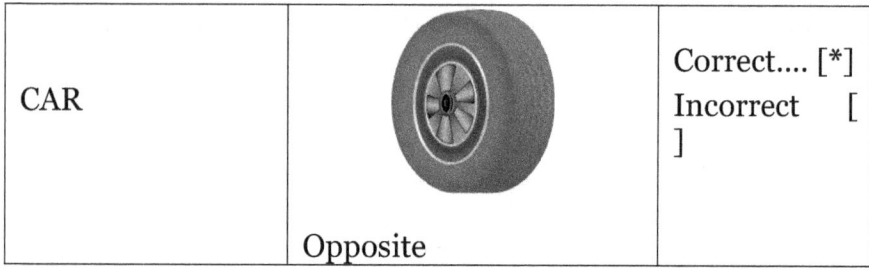 Opposite	Correct.... [*] Incorrect [ ]

The car and tire may be related, but the picture is not exactly the same as the word, so the normal answer would be 'Incorrect'. However since the word opposite appears with the image, the right response is to check 'Correct'

Confused? That's the idea...!

Try this one for yourself before we get going on the full test.

PARCEL	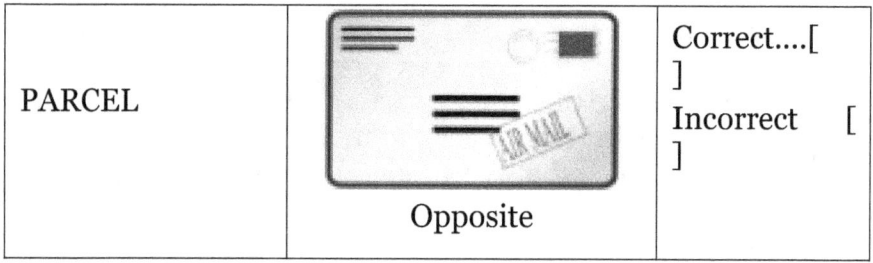 Opposite	Correct....[ ] Incorrect [ ]

What did you select?

The word is **Parcel** but the picture is of a Letter Envelope, so they are not the same. The normal answer then would be 'Incorrect' but because the word 'Opposite' appears with the picture then the true answer to the question is 'Correct'

So grab a pencil and paper, note the time on your watch (you'll need about 60 seconds to complete the test) and let's get started. Write down the question number and your answer.
Remember, the word and the picture must match exactly. But be careful, there's some tricky ones...

1. HONEY		Correct....[ ] Incorrect [ ]
2. SAILBOAT	 Opposite	Correct....[ ] Incorrect [ ]
3. BRIGHT		Correct....[ ] Incorrect [ ]
4. TREE	 Opposite	Correct....[ ] Incorrect [ ]
5. MAN	 Opposite	Correct....[ ] Incorrect [ ]
6. BIRD		Correct....[ ] Incorrect [ ]

7. HOU.S.E	Opposite	Correct....[ ] Incorrect [ ]
8. DOG	Opposite	Correct....[ ] Incorrect [ ]
9. APPLE		Correct....[ ] Incorrect [ ]
10. COW	Opposite	Correct....[ ] Incorrect [ ]

Here are the answers:

1. HONEY		Correct [ ] Incorrect [*]
2. SAILBOAT	Opposite	Correct [ ] Incorrect [*]
3. BRIGHT		Correct [ ] Incorrect.. [*]
4. TREE	Opposite	Correct [ ] Incorrect.. [*]

5. MAN	Opposite	Correct.... [*] Incorrect [ ]
6. BIRD		Correct.... [*] Incorrect [ ]
7. HOU.S.E	Opposite	Correct [ ] Incorrect.. [*]
8. DOG	Opposite	Correct.... [*] Incorrect [ ]
9. APPLE		Correct.... [*] Incorrect [ ]
10. COW	Opposite	Correct.... [*] Incorrect [ ]

Scoring - correct answers:
9 or 10 - You're very accurate
6 to 8 - You were probably going too fast
Under 6 - Maybe you didn't understand the test rules

Timing:
Under 40 seconds, count 5 points:
40 - 60 seconds - count 3 points
Over 1 minute - count 1 point

Now add your two scores together:
14 - 15:   Congratulations you're a quick and accurate thinker
10 - 13:   Quite good but you could improve
9 or less: Your brain speed may be slowing down

So how did you make out in this test? Don't be discouraged if you had a low score, there's lots of reasons:

- you didn't fully understand the quiz
- you were going too quickly
- you weren't concentrating enough
- it was too early in the morning :-)

The 'use it or lose it' rule applies here - the more you can exercise your brain, the more it will improve. As you age your brain naturally slows down. But you can still stay sharp right through your elder years if you make an effort and tackle those mental challenges on a frequent basis.

There are many websites that offer online brain exercises and tests that you can try out. They're fun and I've enjoyed doing them myself. I urge you to check some of them out for yourself. Here's a few to get you started:

Brain Age Games - these are fun and relatively challenging.
http://freebrainagegames.com/

Braingle - this is a standard type of IQ test. It contains 40 questions and takes approximately 30 minutes to complete. I found some of the questions really difficult!
http://www.braingle.com/mind/iq/test.php

Games for the Brain
Lots of choices and some interesting little games
http://www.gamesforthebrain.com/

In conclusion if you want to avoid, or at least slow down, the decline of your mental capacities as you get older, try to get into the habit of following the recommendations in this chapter.

~ ~

Stress Will Kill You - Literally

Stress is your body's response to perceived threatening or demanding situations and it causes mental and physical tension. Under stress your body releases hormones that speed up your system and increase your energy level - a condition often referred to as a fight-or-flight response.

Stress in itself is a normal response. Confronted by a dangerous situation you breathe faster and your pulse rate goes up, sending more oxygen to your brain and other beneficial functions. Even non-threatening settings like being at work with a lot on your work plate can invoke a stressful response in your body.

Stress only becomes bad when it is prolonged, or it happens too frequently. Then it has many serious negative effects including:

- upset stomach
- headaches
- difficulty sleeping
- a weakened immune system

A weakened immune system means you can't fight off infections efficiently. It gets worse - prolonged stress is linked to serious illnesses like heart disease, cancer, liver problems and lung disease. It can lead to depression as well.

So if your plan is to live longer and enjoy your retirement years, it's time to start learning to manage the stress in your life. Nowadays it seems that we face more stressful situations than ever before - the hectic pace of life, financial issues, parents juggling work and family responsibilities and so on. A few lucky people seem to have no problem but most of us struggle with handling stress and we continually worry about everything.

Stress Relief

In my case, constant worry over one thing or another was the principle cause of feeling stressed. Many times it was about things over which I had little control. Fortunately I've since been able to make the distinction and I definitely do not fret over those things I cannot change.

There are lots of medications available to counter the effects of stress, but there are also many things you can do yourself. So unless you are really stressed out in which case see your doctor, you can try the following stress relief tactics.

Identify the causes

What's causing you to feel stressed out all the time? Make a list, include everything you can think of - sometimes it's not one big stressor that is causing the problem but simply a combination of smaller things.

Almost every aspect of our lives can be stressful, if we let it...

- the nature of our work
- our boss at work
- school and college worries
- our family relationships
- our financial situation
- our health
- our weight

Taking stock of everything in your life is a great way to start on a stress reduction plan.

Work on a solution

Be imaginative - write down everything you can possibly think of to eliminate or reduce the cause of the stress. Let's take an example. If you live in a big city as I did in Toronto, driving to work every day can be a constant source of stress. If you find yourself shouting at the driver who cuts in front of you, or you're banging the steering wheel in frustration when you're late and stuck in a traffic jam, then your stress level is increasing (not to mention your blood pressure).

What can you do about it? Well, you could:

- Try public transport - at least for a day or two per week
- Travel with a friend or work colleague sometimes
- You could try to leave earlier in the morning
- Avoid early morning work meetings, if you can
- Is there another less stressful route you could take to work? It may be longer but could be easier on the head
- Are flex work hours available to you? If so you could avoid traveling during prime rush hour times
- Can you work from home? Even just one day a week would break things up

You get the idea... The key here is to stop accepting things the way they are, take a step back and look at the situation more objectively. Maybe you don't have to repeat the daily grind - what about changing jobs or moving closer to work even?

When you realize you <u>can</u> do something about it, stress doesn't have to be a constant part of your life.

Nutrition can help
Do you know that nutrient deficiencies or eating the wrong types of food can increase your stress levels? And eating the right foods can help to lower them.

What we often do is turn to food and drink for emotional relief from stress. So called 'comfort eating' usually means consuming foods that are high in salt, fat or sugar. Things like a few drinks after a hard day, or a late evening binge on ice cream or chocolate are all too common. We tend to crave foods like this because stress increases our cortisol levels.

Cortisol is the hormone that gives you that "fight or flight" feeling when anxiety hits and actually makes you crave your favorite 'comfort food'. The fact is though, these types of food don't help relieve stress and can end up making you feel even more depressed.

What we really need to do is eat the foods that have the opposite effect on your body than stress does. Instead of reaching for the chips try some of these foods that are known for helping your body relieve stress:

- **Blueberries** - high in anti-oxidants, blueberries give your white blood cells a boost and help to counter the effects of stress
- **Dark chocolate** - helps to reduce cortisol levels brought on by stress
- **Nuts and seeds** - sunflower and pumpkin seeds and nuts, especially pistachios, help in the fight against stress
- **Salmon** - has Omega-3 fatty acids helping you to handle stress
- **Turkey** - contains tryptophan, a nutrient that causes your brain to produce the bio-chemical seretonin
- **Spinach** and other dark leafy greens are high in nutrients that help your body produce seretonin and dopamine, both of which help reduce stress

Exercise

As I mentioned before, regular exercise has many benefits and stress reduction is one of them. Stressful situations will always be part of modern living, but exercise makes you much better equipped to handle stress, so that it doesn't take such a heavy toll on you.

How does it work? There are several theories out there. A popular one is that exercise produces endorphins, a brain chemical that produces feelings of well-being. Another theory attributes the stress relief from exercising to the production of another brain chemical called norepinephrine, which helps the brain deal with stress.

Either way, research has definitely shown that exercise relieves stress. So which exercise is best for achieving this goal - hitting a punching bag until your arms feel ready to drop off, or just going for a walk? Actually any type of exercise between these two extremes will work. Personally I like running because you can take it easy or you can pick up the pace and go for a harder workout if you feel like it.

The bottom line is simply to do something active - don't just sit on the couch feeling miserable or worried.

Meditation

Practicing meditation is a simple and effective way to combat stress. You can meditate anywhere - you don't have to be lying on a bed in a darkened room. You could be out for a walk, sitting at your desk, or even be in a meeting!

How does meditation help reduce stress? When we meditate, our body starts to relax; we breathe more slowly and our pulse rate goes down. In fact we are achieving a state that is opposite of the 'fight or flight' response generated by stressful situations. Although it's not a common technique in the Western world, meditation is something anyone can learn to do quite easily. Eastern cultures have practiced this technique for thousands of years as a way of achieving inner peace and enlightenment.

There are several different types of meditation but they are all designed to achieve the same goals:

- Relax your body
- Clear your mind

For example one method requires you to focus your mind on how your body feels in the moment - your breathing, your heart beat, the feeling in your arms, legs and feet. If you do this for just a few moments you'll find that you are much calmer, your brain has slowed down and you're no longer consumed by worrisome, troubled thoughts.

Another variation of the above technique, is to say a word or phrase (called a mantra) to yourself over and over so that no other thoughts intrude on your conscious mind. The phrase should be calming like "I feel relaxed" or inspirational like "believe".

Yoga
Yoga is another great way to fight stress. Originating from Asia, this mind-body discipline combines exercise and meditation to achieve complete relaxation. Yoga uses physical poses, controlled breathing and meditation. If you do this regularly, or even better, join a Yoga class, you will be more relaxed generally and better able to manage stress.

My Experience
I'd never tried meditating until just a few years ago and was surprised to find how well it worked. Whenever I have problems falling asleep at night, I do a meditation routine and I usually fall asleep in no time.

~~~~~~~~~~~~~~~~~~~~~~~

Sleep

Sleep plays such an important part in our mental and physical well being that I've devoted a full chapter to this topic. I didn't always get eight hours sleep per night as I do now. In fact as a young man, like many of my peers I thought sleep was almost a waste of time - I'd rather be awake doing something else. This was completely wrong and I would have performed much better and achieved more if I'd started going to bed earlier every night.

Benjamin Franklin is quoted as saying *"Early to bed and early to rise, makes a man healthy, wealthy and wise"*. Did they know back then in the 1700's the importance of sleep? I'm not sure about the 'wealthy' part, but getting enough sleep is certainly necessary for your overall health and wellness and your brain! Many studies have been conducted to determine the benefits we get from a proper night's sleep. These include:

- Reduced stress
- Improved mood
- Improved learning ability
- Repairing your heart and blood vessels.
- Maintaining a healthy balance of the hormones that control your eating
- Helping your immune system to stay healthy.
- Helping you function well throughout the day

How much do we need?
Nowadays the accepted number of hours sleep we need is 7-8 hours per night for most people (a small percentage of the population can get by on less). But how many of us actually get to enjoy that amount? If you don't then you're not alone - 40% of Americans sleep less than the recommended amount. The secret is going to sleep about 7.5 hours before you have to get up in the morning. This probably means 8 hours, since you may not go to sleep as soon as you get to bed.

Problems of Insufficient Sleep

If you constantly get less sleep you run a greater risk of heart and kidney disease, high blood pressure, diabetes and stroke. You will feel drowsy at points during the day and have a slower reaction time.

> *Studies have shown that the number of accidents due to lack of sleep is comparable to those from drunk driving.*

When I was in my thirties and forties I often got by on six hours or less of sleep on several days of the week. It was only when I took up regular running that I found I really needed to sleep more. Daily exercise is a great way to encourage a good night's sleep. It's also strongly recommended not to watch TV in bed, nor read your tablet or smart phone.

Your Daily Schedule

I found my schedule was the biggest obstacle to getting enough sleep. I was always an early riser and when I lived in the Midwest, I'd be up by 5:30 AM every weekday. So I gradually got into the habit of going to bed early. It took some doing at first, since I liked watching the late night TV shows. Instead of TV I now read a book at bedtime and I usually fall asleep by 10:30 PM every night. I've been doing that now for many years and I'm convinced it's one of the key factors that contributes to my good health.

Sleep and Stress

Too much stress causes you to sleep poorly and a lack of sleep increases stress. It's a downhill spiral to ill health that you need to avoid at all costs. How often do we lay awake in bed thinking about things that prevent us from falling asleep. This can happen when you first go to bed or if you wake up in the middle of the night.

One thing I've noticed is that everything seems larger than life in the middle of the night. Noises are louder, and our worries are definitely bigger. But then you wake up the next morning and wonder why you were so stressed about something or other. If you can capture that morning feeling you'll get back to sleep easier.

Tips to get to sleep

- I've found that reading a book when I first go to bed helps me fall asleep right away. This is counter-intuitive because you would expect that what you had just been reading would keep you awake.

- If I wake up in the night and find my thoughts are stopping me from getting back to sleep, I practice one of the meditation techniques I described in the previous chapter and that usually works.

- Don't look at the clock - that only makes things worse

- If you really cannot fall asleep, get up and read a book

Before you go to bed...

Here are some things you can do before bedtime that will set you up for a better night's sleep:

- Try to go to bed at the same time every night. Your body will get used to the routine and you'll naturally feel tired as bed time approaches

- Make sure the room is dark

- Use a comfortable mattress and find a pillow that's right for you

- Keep your bedroom cool if you can. A good temperature is 68° F (20° C) or even less if you prefer. I find it's a trade-off between the coolness of the room and needing too many bed covers

- Have a soothing tea before you retire at night. I have a chamomile tea every evening and find that it helps me relax, which is always a good precursor to a sound night's sleep

- Try to avoid eating at least three hours before you go to bed

- Don't have too much alcohol. You might fall asleep quickly but you'll almost certainly wake up later on

- Avoid caffeine (coffee, black tea and chocolate for example)

Exercise

As I've said many times throughout this book, exercise is good for you and this includes helping you sleep soundly. If you've exercised during the day, your body will naturally want to recover and you'll find it easier to get to sleep. Another effective habit to promote sleep is to go for a walk after dinner. I used to do this when we owned a dog, but unfortunately I've lost the routine.

Medications to help you sleep?

As a last resort you may be considering taking meds to help you sleep better. If you are suffering from insomnia and just cannot get a good night's rest you need to see your doctor. He may be able to identify the cause and treat it instead of prescribing a sleeping pill.

I'm certainly not a fan of using prescription drugs to alleviate sleeping disorders - many of the meds are addictive and have side effects. Besides, the real issue is to find out why you are not sleeping properly. This is a major problem you have to solve or else your health will definitely suffer in the long term.

What about the over-the-counter sleep aids that are very popular? Again this wouldn't be my first choice and I'd rather see my doctor first anyway. You can actually build up a resistance to some of the products that contain antihistamines and they become less effective with continued use.

Natural Cures

There are several natural herbs that are supposed to help with sleeping problems:

- **Tart Cherry Juice** - contains Tryptophan, an essential amino acid that causes our bodies to produce melatonin. Melatonin is a bio-chemical that regulates our sleep-wake cycle and promotes drowsiness when we go to bed.

- **Valerian root** - typically taken as a tea.

- **Melatonin supplement** - not strictly natural, since it's sold in synthetic form. A popular use is to help you recover from jet lag.

- **Chamomile** - as I mentioned above, this herb, taken as a tea, has soothing qualities that can help us relax and sleep better.

I would definitely try these natural cures before taking prescription drugs. The problem is that there's not much scientific evidence showing that they are effective treatments. Research on tart cherry juice has shown positive results, so it's at the top of my list.

Bottom Line...

If you're not sleeping very well or waking up frequently during the night don't just accept this as a given. You can (and should) start do something about it. Proper sleep is so important to all aspects of wellness it's not something to ignore if you want to live a longer healthier life.

~~~~~~~~~~~~~~~~~~~~~

Section IV Highlights & Summary

Following are some of the key points covered in this section about the strong influence your mind has over your body.

Mental Fitness

Mental fitness is just as important as physical fitness when it comes to your overall health and well being. Eastern civilizations have always stressed the importance of the mental side of life and our inner connection to each other and the world.

Neuroplasticity

Modern science has shown that your brain has the ability to modify itself. Previously, it was thought that the brain stopped developing in adolescence and the connections that were formed between the brain cells were fixed and stayed that way as we aged. Now we know this is not the case. Your brain has the ability to change even in older years, - it can re-organize pathways and create new connections.

Motivation

Without enough motivation, you're not likely to achieve anything. Yet many people seem to lack motivation and they go through life on auto-pilot, without any real appreciation or enjoyment. Each of us needs to motivate ourselves, given the right environment and goals, in order to achieve what we want.

Brain Health

One of our biggest worries about getting older is a reduction in our mental capacity. But there's a lot we can do to slow down or even prevent this from happening. Your brain benefits from use. Since our brain and body are intricately connected, exercising the body is good for the brain and doing mental exercises to improve brain health is also good for the body.

The Importance of A Healthy Brain

Why is your brain health so important? Your brain is responsible for the production of many hormones and bio-chemicals that have a profound effect on the health and aging of your body. The faster your brain ages - the older you will look and feel. Your cognitive abilities will also start to be impaired.

Brain Exercises

Get into the habit of exercising your brain in different ways by doing things like crossword puzzles, Sudoku and brain teasers.

Nutrition Helps

Eating the right foods can play an important role in keeping your brain healthy.

Reduce sugary foods, (except natural fruit) - sugar is bad for you and has a negative effect on brain function. It can also contribute to brain shrinkage.

Omega-3 fatty acids and blueberries help protect the brain and slow down memory loss associated with aging.

SECTION V - The Inside Story

"The quality, not the longevity, of one's life is what is important" - Martin Luther King, Jr.

This section looks at two important factors affecting our wellness - our blood and our genetic makeup. I discuss the question of how much do they influence the state of our health and the rate of aging?

Am I Missing Something?

Like many of us I wonder about the proper levels of nutrients in my body. Even if we eat fairly healthy meals, there's still a chance we could have low levels of some key vitamin or mineral. The huge supplements industry relies on this uncertainty to sell North Americans more than $30 billion of nutritional and vitamin supplements every year.

There are literally hundreds of blood tests available that measure everything from cell counts to zinc levels. The question is - are these tests effective and do they provide any meaningful information?

Following are just some of the common blood tests available:

- **Glucose Level:** Measures the risk of developing diabetes. This test claims to be able to predict diabetes (glucose level over 120), many years before it actually happens. Another good test is **A1C** that measures the amount of hemoglobin in the blood that has glucose attached to it. This test measures average blood glucose amounts over the previous 2 - 3 months.

- **HDL/LDL:** cholesterol test. LDL is the 'bad' cholesterol, which in excess, can lead to the build up of plaque on artery walls. HDL is known as the "good cholesterol" - it removes the LDL type.

- **Triglycerides:** Stored fats used by the body to provide energy. However elevated triglyceride levels increase the risk of stroke, heart attack, heart disease and other serious health issues.

- **Complete Blood Count:** This is not a definitive diagnostic test, but is often used to indicate or confirm other problems. The complete blood count measures the concentrations of red and white blood cells, hemoglobin and platelets in your blood.

- **C-reactive protein (CRP):** Increased levels of this protein in your blood indicate the presence of inflammation in your body. This could be a sign of narrowing of the arteries in your heart.

- **CO2 Level:** This test, along with the next three (chloride, potassium and sodium) are all part of your blood's Electrolytes analysis. Carbon dioxide levels measure the pH or acid/alkaline balance in the tissues.

- **Chloride:** This electrolyte helps to maintain an acid/alkaline balance. Abnormal levels can indicate heart, kidney, liver issues and high blood pressure.

- **Potassium:** Proper levels of potassium are necessary for the correct functioning of your heart, muscles and nerves. Abnormal levels can lead to heart issues like an irregular heartbeat.

- **Sodium:** Measures the salt / water balance in your body. A level that is too low may indicate heart or kidney problems. A high level is indicative of a diet too high in salt or insufficient water.

- **Magnesium:** This mineral is used in almost all the chemical processes in your body. Magnesium also helps regulate blood pressure and keeps your heart functioning.

- **Serum Iron:** Iron is essential to making hemoglobin in the blood and to help transfer oxygen to the muscle. If your iron level is too low your muscles will not perform at their best.

- **Omega-3 - omega 6**: Most people in north America have levels of omega-3 fatty acids that are too low and omega-6 levels that are too high.

- **Vitamin D** - this essential vitamin is often too low in many people. The test to measure the amount in your blood is called a 25(OH)D test.

- **Vitamin B12** - another important vitamin that becomes harder to absorb as we age.

To answer my question above, are the tests accurate? Well, I think most of them are, provided you carefully follow the pre-test instructions. For example many of the tests require 12 hours fasting prior to the test.

Tests for vitamin D levels are somewhat controversial and results are reportedly wrong or inconsistent. Naturally the leading companies involved defend their tests, claiming they do provide valid results. Check with your health care professional on this one.

~ ~ ~ ~ ~ ~ ~ ~ ~ ~ ~ ~ ~ ~ ~ ~ ~ ~ ~ ~

Genes and the Human Genome

I'm including this chapter because there is an enormous amount of genetic research underway and it's important for us to be familiar with the basic concepts of genetics so we understand what the science refers to when it comes to DNA, genes and chromosomes.

Current research is revealing important insights into how our genes affect our health and aging. I'm convinced that this research will prove that a lot of what we know empirically about the effect of diet and exercise on our health will be true.

I expect we'll be hearing more and more about this topic as time goes on. I believe we'll soon be at the stage where everyone will have a routine genetic analysis done, just like the blood tests we go for on a regular basis now.

To help you understand the terminology, here is my very elementary explanation of the relationship between DNA, genes and chromosomes.

DNA

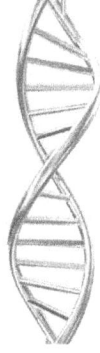 You've probably seen this picture, or something similar before. Called a double helix, it represents a strand of our DNA (deoxyribonucleic acid), the basic building block of our cells. This helix model was developed by Nobel prize winners James Watson and Francis Crick in the 1950s. However DNA itself was first discovered way back in 1863 by Friedrich Miescher a Swiss physician and medical researcher.

DNA is found in the nucleus of every cell of our body, except for the red blood cells. It is the fundamental unit of our genetic material. Each DNA molecule contains four types of nitrogen bases, commonly known by their initials A, T, G and C. The order of these bases determines our DNA's instructions, or genetic code.

The actual structure of a molecule of DNA is such that there are an infinite number of ways that it can be put together, accounting for all the different species on earth. Minor differences in genetic make-up mean a lot! For example the DNA of humans and chimpanzees is 99% identical.

The amazing thing about our DNA is that although all humans share between 99 to 99.9% identical DNA among themselves, the remaining one percent or less contains enough minor variations to make each one of us uniquely different from the other.

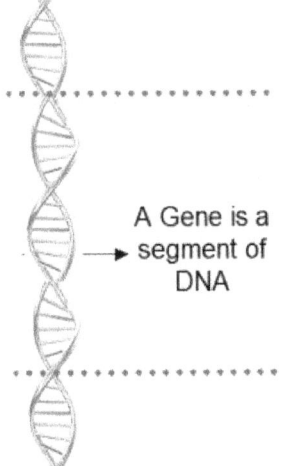

Genes

A Gene is a segment of DNA

Genes are segments of our DNA structure and represent the blueprint for our biological makeup. Genes contain the instructions for producing proteins that determine our physical characteristics - everything from the color of our eyes to the size of our feet. We have about 25,000 different genes in our body.

The interesting thing about genes is that they are not always active in our cells. They can be turned on or off by external factors like our diet, chemical exposure, exercise and aging, or by messages from other genes. This messaging ability is a very important attribute of our genes, as it can have a direct influence on the state of our health. I'll mention this again in more detail in the section on Epigenetics - the study of how genes are switched on or off.

Chromosomes

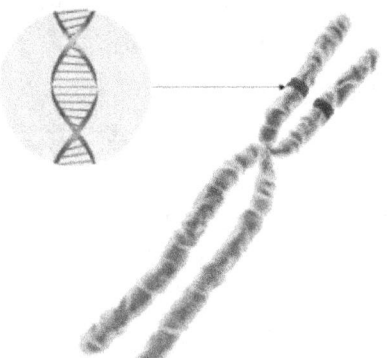

Chromosomes are strands of DNA packed in tightly wound structures, that allow long strings of DNA to fit inside a cell's nucleus. Chromosomes are present in all of our cells (except for red blood cells that do not have a nucleus).

We all have 46 chromosomes, grouped into 23 pairs. The chromosome is a way of getting all of the DNA information into every cell into our body. This allows for cell division - necessary for growth and functioning - to occur.

So to summarize the relationships between these elements we have:

DNA >> Genes >> Chromosomes

To further help us understand this relationship, a popular analogy uses a city as a comparison. Think of each DNA molecule as a single house. A gene would be a street of houses. A neighborhood that contains several streets represents a chromosome. Finally a city containing several neighborhoods would be a set of chromosomes that determine a particular species such as humans.

The Human Genome Project

The Human Genome Project was an international scientific research project with the goal of determining the sequence of chemical base pairs which make up human DNA and of identifying and mapping all of the genes of the human genome from both a physical and a functional standpoint. It began in 1990 and was completed in 2003. The human genome was the first of all vertebrates to be sequenced and was completed in 2001. Since then thousands of human genomes have been completely sequenced and many more have been mapped at lower levels of resolution.

Genome sequencing is the first step in deciphering the genetic code of a species. It helps understand how the complete genome works and how various genes work together in managing the growth, development and functioning of an organism.

Today there are several companies that offer genomic analysis for individuals. They provide information on inherited conditions for certain diseases, responses to drugs, genetic risk factors, ancestry and more.

~~~~~~~~~~~~~~~~~~~~~~

Do Your Genes Contain The Final Answer?

There's a strong belief held by many people, including some traditional medical practitioners and scientists, that our future health and aging is pre-determined by our genes. The argument then goes on to say that our risk of succumbing to an inherited disease is much greater than for people who do not carry that gene.

Some genetic scientists have even proposed that it's not only our health and longevity that are written in our genes, but our whole personality as well. The implications are disturbing - does that mean a person may be born a criminal instead of becoming one?

Lifestyle or Genes?

This popular argument poses the question - which is more important in deciding our health, is it our inherited genetic make up or is it our lifestyle? I've always believed that our lifestyle was just as important as our genetic traits in determining our health, wellness and longevity. If you knew you had a pre-disposition to cancer for example then you could adjust your diet accordingly and start exercising to reduce the risk of contracting the disease. The idea that preventing cancer can be achieved by lifestyle changes used to be discredited by mainstream medical science, but this is beginning to change. Institutions like Cancer Research UK say " ... experts estimate that more than 4 in 10 cancer cases could be prevented by lifestyle changes".

It's not clear to me why only 40% of cases - why not more? When you look at the alternative chronic disease treatments available today (many of which are only found outside of the U.S.A and Canada) there are lots of cures that rely more on dietary changes than any other method. However there are only a few published research study results of these treatments and I've yet to see any statistics about the success rates of such cures.

Epigenetics
This relatively new field of genetics is the study of biological processes that can switch genes off and on. What does that mean? Well, in theory, we could turn off the 'bad' genes and prevent cancer and other chronic diseases, slow down the aging process and lots more.

Still in the research stages, epigenetics does seem to prove that the genes we are born with won't automatically lead to ill health, Alzheimer's, or premature aging.

So my personal answer to the question in the chapter heading, 'Do Your Genes Contain The Final Answer?' is - yes they may, but only if you don't do anything about it and just let it happen!

~~~~~~~~~~~~~~~~~~~~

Section V Highlights & Summary

Nutrient Levels
Many of us wonder if we getting the proper amounts of nutrients in our body. The huge supplements industry relies on this uncertainty to sell us more than $30 billion of supplements every year.

Blood Analyses
There are literally hundreds of blood tests available that measure everything from cell counts to zinc levels. Some of these are more accurate than others.

Genetics
This science is advancing quickly and I expect we'll soon be getting regular genetic analyses done as part of our health check-ups.

DNA, Genes & Chromosomes
DNA is found in the nucleus of every cell of our body, except for the red blood cells. It is the fundamental unit of our genetic material. Genes are segments of our DNA structure and represent the blueprint for our biological makeup.
Chromosomes are strands of DNA that allow long strings of DNA to fit inside a cell's nucleus. We all have 46 chromosomes, grouped into 23 pairs.

The Human Genome Project
The Human Genome Project was completed in 2003. It was an international scientific research project with the goal of mapping all of the genes that make up the human genome.

Is lifestyle or genetic make-up more important to our health?
Epigenetics, a relatively new branch of genetics, seems to prove that the genes we are born with won't automatically lead to ill health, Alzheimer's, or premature aging.

SECTION VI - Live Better, Live Longer

"God gave us the gift of life; it is up to us to give ourselves the gift of living well." - Voltaire

This is where it all comes together and we look at what I did, and what you need to start doing if you want to improve your chances for a healthy future and a longer, more enjoyable life.

You're Never Old Until...

Most people in their forties and early fifties don't worry too much about getting old - that's something that happens when you're seventy and over, right? Well, the decline in our health often starts in our forties or even earlier. We don't get old overnight, it just creeps up on us little by little, day by day, so we barely notice it. However there are several signs that you may not be as young as you used to be. Here's some warning signals to watch out for as you reach the next decade in your life.

The Forties

For women this is often the period when weight gain occurs and a few wrinkles start showing up. This is the time when you look more critically at your face in the mirror. For men, weight around the middle becomes a problem and it's hard to lose. The probability of an enlarged prostate gland also becomes more common.

Increased stress levels are common in this age group and if you read the chapter on stress you know how this can be setting the stage for future health problems to occur.

You may also start to experience some chronic pain in your back and joints and this can become worse as you get into your next decade.

The Fifties

Women generally reach menopause at this time and as their hormone levels change they may also become more susceptible to heart disease and osteoporosis. The risk of breast cancer also increases during this period. Men may begin to experience some erectile dysfunction issues during their fifties.

For both sexes, digestive problems may start to show up during this time, partially caused by lower levels of beneficial bacteria in your gut.

Your memory may also not be as good as it was and your ability to accurately recall events declines.

The Sixties

Many people may start to suffer from reduced hearing in their sixties. Eye problems that started in the previous decade, become more apparent. Macular degeneration - a deterioration of the central portion of the retina - is more common and affects more than 10 million north Americans.

Bone health can start to decline and osteoporosis becomes a common problem. Joint pain that started earlier in life becomes worse as arthritis sets in. Bladder control too becomes an issue, especially in people over 65.

Do you have any of these symptoms? If you do it's time to see your health professional, especially when it comes to your eyesight. For example, macular degeneration can be treated if it's caught early enough.

Now I didn't put these age-related health concerns in just to scare you and hopefully you don't have any of the issues associated with your age group. Sometimes however there are subtle indications that you notice about yourself and you should try to resolve them, even if it's just a precaution.

At the age of seventy six, apart from looking older and having less hair, I don't have any of the above health problems (so far!) and I want you to take that as an encouragement. If you begin living healthier earlier on in your life (as I did) you could significantly reduce the risks of suffering from these common health issues. By starting to improve your lifestyle as soon as you can, you will also reduce your risk of developing serious problems like diabetes, cancer and heart disease later on in your life.

Real age vs. Actual age

I referred to this idea earlier in the chapter on Brain Health. Our bodies age due to cellular damage associated with such factors as genetics, lifestyle and environment. The more damage that occurs the older we look and feel compared to our actual, or chronological, age. The following graph illustrates this concept. For example if your actual age was 65 your real, or physical, age could vary by plus or minus seven years (58 to 72) in this hypothetical case.

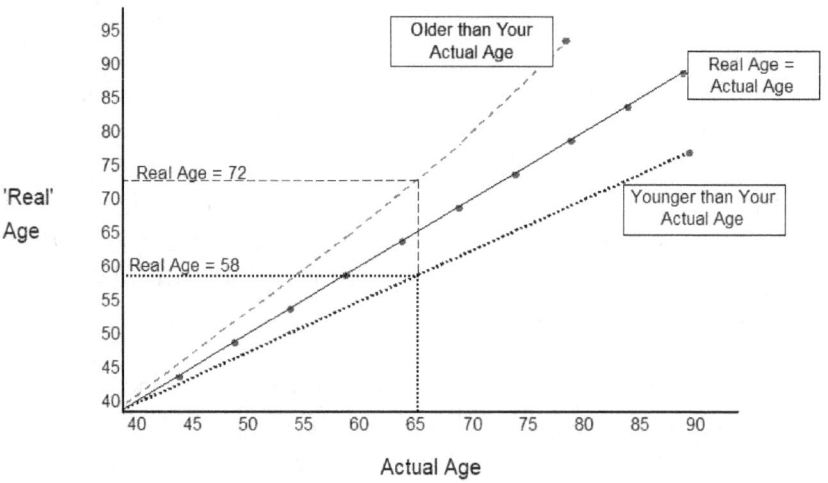

Naturally everyone is different and there are many ways and tests you can use to figure out how well you are aging. Just Google "Real age tests" and you'll get a couple pages of results showing different tests. According to an article on the website webmd.com, "A simple urine test apparently can reveal how old your body really is - showing its biological, not chronological age".

Are these tests very accurate? Personally I doubt it, but they probably do give a reasonable estimate of how you are doing (compared to an 'average' person). Actually I just ask my doctor after completing my annual physical check-up and he's able to make a good assessment of my physical age.

~~~~~~~~~~~~~~~~~~~~~

Wellness Self-Assessment

The GPS in your car would be useless at guiding you anywhere if it didn't know exactly where it was to start with. Likewise, before you start setting goals and making lifestyle changes to improve your wellness level you need to know where you are at today. To help you do this, I've put together a self assessment questionnaire for you to complete.

♥ Health Hint

Although I've called this chapter *Self* Assessment if you haven't had a doctor's check-up, including blood work analysis, within the last year or so I strongly suggest you do this first. In fact if you're over 50 you should be getting regular yearly check-ups anyway.

The Wellness Questionnaire

This covers some of the important aspects of wellness, based on the definition I presented in section I.

"Wellness is a state of complete physical, mental and social well-being and not merely the absence of disease or infirmity."

The following questions cover five main components of wellness:

1. Nutrition
2. Fitness
3. Stress Levels
4. General Health
5. Brain Health

There are almost 100 questions and it will take you about 15 - 20 minutes to complete. Don't worry too much about your final score (although you may want to check with your health professional if it's really low!).

One important benefit you'll get from completing the test is the fact that you've taken a systematic review of your own wellness level.

Important Note

> *This test is only intended to give you an idea where you could be on the wellness scale. It is not a substitute for a complete analysis and assessment by a health professional.*

Instructions:

For each question, circle the answer that best applies to you. *If you're reading this as an eBook take a piece of paper and jot down your selection to each question (e.g. 1B, 2C, 3B, etc).* When you complete all the questions in a section, total up the number of A, B and C answers and enter the count in the table at the end of that section. The final scoring and assessment for each Wellness category can be found at the end of the test.

Note:

This is a long test but I encourage you to work your way through it. You don't need to do it all in one go either. It's worth the effort as I'm sure you'll find the results quite revealing.

Part I: Nutrition

How well do you eat, compared to current nutritional guidelines?

#	Nutrition Question	A	B	C
1.	How often do you eat fresh fruit?	Every Day	3-4 times per week	Less than 3 times

#	Nutrition Question	A	B	C
2.	How often do you eat fresh vegetables like broccoli, carrots, cauliflower etc.,	Every Day	3 -4 times per week	Less than 3 times
3.	Do you eat many salads?	4 - 7 times per week	2 - 3 times weekly	Less than 2 times
4.	Do you eat foods like sweet potato or squash?	2 - 3 times per week	1 - 2 times per week	Rarely
5.	Do you eat nuts and seeds, including almonds and walnuts?	3 - 5 times per week	1 - 2 times per week	Rarely
6a or 6b	Do you eat much coldwater fish (salmon, cod etc.)? *For vegans & vegetarians who eat no fish or animal-based products* Are you taking a DHA supplement?	2 or more times per week At least 3 or more times per week	Once a week 1 - 2 times per week	Rarely No
7.	Do you ever eat meatless dinners like Greek salad, vegetable pizza or stew?	3 times or more times per week	1 or 2 times weekly	Rarely
8.	Do you eat whole grain (i.e. not white) breads, cereals, pasta, rice etc?	Always	Mostly	Rarely - I prefer white bread
9.	How often to you eat red meats, like beef, pork or lamb?	2 times per week or less	3 - 4 times per week	5 - 7 times per week
10.	How often do you eat fast food meals?	Once a week or less	2 - 3 times per week	4 times or more per week
11.	How often do you have frozen dinners, including pizza?	Once a week or less	2 - 3 times per week	4 times or more per week

#	Nutrition Question	A	B	C
12.	How many times per week do you have dinner out, or order in meals from restaurants?	1- 2 times per week or less	3 - 4 times per week	More than 4 times
13.	How often do you eat sweet foods like donuts, cookies, chocolate and candy	Rarely	Sometimes	Often, almost every day
14.	How many alcoholic drinks do you consume each day?	2 or less per day, on most days	3 - 4 per day	More than 4 drinks daily
15.	How many sodas or sports drinks do you consume each day?	One a day, or less	2 - 3 per day	4 or more daily

Nutrition Count:

A's	B's	C's

Part II: Fitness

'Fitness' is an elusive term and not easy to define precisely. Here we are referring to your body composition and your general ability to get around and easily perform regular daily activities.

#	Fitness Question	A	B	C
1.	Can you climb a flight of stairs without feeling out of breath?	Yes	I'm breathing a little harder	I'm out of breath by the time I reach the top
2.	Can you get in and out of your car easily, without any pain	Always	Mostly	No, it's a bit of a struggle
3.	Are you overweight? Check the weight table below	I'm in the correct weight range	I'm overweight	I'm obese
4.	Do you exercise regularly?	4 or more days per week,	2 - 3 days	1 day or less per week
5.	Do you include both aerobic exercise such as jogging and anaerobic exercise like strength training, in your weekly workouts?	Yes - I do both types of exercise during the week	Sometimes	I don't work out regularly at all
6.	Do you have difficulty lifting and carrying weights like heavy shopping bags?	No, I'm quite strong	Sometimes	Yes - I usually need help

#	Fitness Question	A	B	C
7.	How many sit-ups (crunches) can you do from a lying down position without straining?	60 or more	20 - 60	Less than 20
8.	Can you touch your toes without bending your knees	Yes - no problem	Almost!	No, I can't
9.	How many hours a day do you spend sitting down?	5 hours or less	6 -10 hours	More than 10 hours
10.	Is your blood pressure in the recommended range? (See below for normal readings)	Yes - I'm OK	Up to 10 points higher than the normal for my age	More than 10 points over normal
11.	Take your pulse rate (See below on how to take your pulse)	Between 45 and 65 beats per minute	66 - 80	Over 80
12.	Do you get tired easily after physical exertion or being on your feet for long?	No	I do start to feel tired after an hour or so	I seem to tire easily if I'm doing any physical work
13.	On a scale of 1 (low) to 10 (high) how positive and energetic do you usually feel?	8 -10	5 - 7	4 or less
14.	How's your appetite?	Good - I eat well	Good most of the time, but not always	Not great, I often leave food on my plate

#	Fitness Question	A	B	C
15.	Do you have regular bowel movements?	Yes	Most of the time	No and I sometimes suffer from constipation

Fitness Count:

A's	B's	C's

Average Weight Table:

The average weight in pounds is given for your height and body frame type.

Height	Women			Men		
	Small frame	Medium frame	Large frame	Small frame	Medium frame	Large frame
4' 10"	102-111	109-121	118-131			
4' 11"	103-113	111-123	120-134			
5' 0"	104-115	113-126	122-137			
5' 1"	106-118	115-129	125-140			
5' 2"	108-121	118-132	128-143	128-134	131-141	138-150
5' 3"	111-124	121-135	131-147	130-136	133-143	140-153
5' 4"	114-127	124-138	134-151	132-138	135-145	142-156
5' 5"	117-130	127-141	137-155	134-140	137-148	144-160
5' 6"	120-133	130-144	140-159	136-142	139-151	146-164
5' 7"	123-136	133-147	143-163	138-145	142-154	149-168
5' 8"	126-139	136-150	146-167	140-148	145-157	152-172
5' 9"	129-142	139-153	149-170	142-151	148-160	155-176
5' 10"	132-145	142-156	152-173	144-154	151-163	158-180
5' 11"	135-148	145-159	155-176	146-157	154-166	161-184
6' 0"	138-151	148-162	158-179	149-160	157-170	164-188
6' 1"				152-164	160-174	168-192
6' 2"				155-168	164-178	172-197

| Height | Women | | | Men | | |
	Small frame	Medium frame	Large frame	Small frame	Medium frame	Large frame
6' 3"				158-172	167-182	176-202
6' 4"				162-176	171-187	181-207

Taking your Pulse:

1. Take your pulse on the inside of your wrist, just below the thumb.
2. Using the tips of your first two fingers press gently on the blood vessels on your wrist.
3. Count your pulse for 10 seconds and then multiply by 6 to find the number of beats per minute.

Recommended Blood Pressure:

Normal blood pressure is between **110/75** on the low end to **130/85** on the high side. As we get older our blood pressure readings tend to increase. Here are some average readings:

Age	Blood Pressure
45-49	127/84
50-54	129/85
55-59	131/86
60+	134/87

Your blood pressure will also vary a lot during the day. I have a simple home blood pressure monitor and I find my blood pressure is lower in the morning and higher later on in the afternoon. You also need to take two or three readings at a time and take the average for a more accurate result.

Part III Stress Level

Note: if you are retired or do not work just answer the work-related questions with an 'A' score.

#	Question	A	B	C
1.	Are you working or retired?	Retired more than a year	Retired less than one year	I'm working
2.	Do you live in a big city?	No - I live in a small town or rural	Mid - size city	Yes
3.	Do you drive to work in heavy traffic	No	Moderate traffic	Yes
4.	Do you interact with the public as part of your work?	Rarely or never	Sometimes	Yes
5.	Does your work involve meeting frequent deadlines, multi-tasking or working in a competitive environment	Rarely or never	Sometimes	Yes
6.	Do you often have to work overtime?	Rarely or never	Sometimes	Yes
7.	How much sleep do you usually get?	7 - 8 hours	6 - 7 hours	Less than 6
8.	Do you often wake up during the night and then have difficulty getting back to sleep?	Rarely	Sometimes	Often
9.	Do you find yourself worrying a lot?	Rarely	Sometimes	Often
10.	Are you often edgy and irritable?	Rarely	Sometimes	Often

#	Question	A	B	C
11.	Do you exercise regularly?	More than 4 times per week	3 or 4 times per week	No - less than twice a week
12.	Are you drinking more alcohol than you used to?	No	A little more	Yes - quite a bit
13.	Do you suffer from loss of appetite, or do you sometimes over-indulge when it comes to food	Rarely or never	Sometimes	Yes
14.	Are you experiencing family or relationship issues and conflict?	Rarely or never	Sometimes	Yes
15.	Have there been any major changes in your life such as death of a loved one, new job, or relocation	No	Minor changes	Yes

Stress Level Count:

A's	B's	C's

Part IV General health

This part of the questionnaire assesses the general state of your overall health. **It's an indication only,** there are so many factors that can affect your health we'd need a multi-page questionnaire to cover them all.

* *It is not meant as a substitute for a proper checkup from your doctor.*

Even if you have a top score, you could still have a health problem, so confirm the results with a follow-up visit to your health professional.

#	Question	A	B	C
1.	Do you regularly take any prescription medications?	None	1 -2 per day	Three or more
2.	Do you have any of the following conditions: Cardiovascular disease, Arthritis, Diabetes, Cancer or Lung disease?	None	I have one of the conditions listed, but not advanced	I have two or more and /or I have one that is in an advanced state
3.	Do you have high cholesterol?	No	Somewhat high	Yes
4.	How is your Blood Pressure ? (see the table above in the Fitness section)	In the normal range for my age	Slightly higher than normal	High - over 140/90
5.	How often do you catch a cold or flu'?	Once every two years, or less frequently	about once per year	Two or more times each year

#	Question	A	B	C
6.	How active are you on a daily basis?	I move around a lot, or I work out	I do some physical activity daily	I do very little
7.	How do you feel physically?	Good, for the majority of the time	Some days I don't feel so good	I often don't feel well
8.	How's your appetite?	Good - I always enjoy my meals	It's OK - but sometimes I'm not hungry at mealtimes	Poor, I often have to force myself to finish dinner
9.	Do you suffer from joint pain?	Not at all	Sometimes	Frequently
10.	Do you have any restricted motion, e.g. in your shoulder or legs?	Not at all	A little	Yes, I just can't move as well as before
11.	Are you overweight?	No	Somewhat	Yes
12.	What's your general outlook on life?	Positive	Up and down - it depends...	Mostly negative, I'm rarely optimistic
13.	Do you smoke?	No		Yes
14.	Did you score more than 20 on the Stress section of this assessment?	Yes		No
15.	Do you have any family history of cardiovascular problems?	No		Yes

General Health Count:

A's	B's	C's

Part V Brain Health

Brain health is an important part of wellness. As we reach middle age and beyond we all tend to become more forgetful.

Brain Health General Questions:

#	Question	A	B	C
1.	Check your **Brain Age** test score from the Brain Health chapter in Section IV and select the column A, B or C that applies to your score	21 - 25	14 - 20	13 or less
2.	How often do you misplace everyday items like car keys, eyeglasses, etc?	Rarely	Sometimes	Often
3.	Do you do regular aerobic exercises like jogging, cycling or brisk walking?	4 or more times per week	2 - 3 times per week	Rarely
4.	Do you ever forget the name of someone you know when you meet them?	Occasionally	From time to time	Often
5.	Does your memory seem a lot worse than it used to be?	No, it's about the same	Somewhat worse	A lot worse, I'm forgetting things often
6.	Do you have a problem learning new things, like how to use a new cell phone, or play a new card game	No - I learn easily	Sometimes - it depends what it is	Quite often

#	Question	A	B	C
7.	Do you ever play games like Sudoku, or do crossword puzzles or brain teasers?	Often - most days	Sometimes - 2 or 3 times per week	Rarely

Brain health Count:

A's	B's	C's

Full Wellness Test Scoring

Now refer back to the table totals you completed at the end of each part of the test. You'll count 3 points for every answer you chose in column A, 2 for every one in column B and zero for answers in column C.

Enter your column counts in the tables below and add up the total.

1. Nutrition

Column	Count	Value	Score
A's		x 3	
B's		x 2	
C's		x 0	
-	-	**Total...**	

Assessment:

- If you scored **40 - 45** you're eating really well and your overall health should benefit.

- If you have **30 - 39** this is still quite good, but you could make some healthier choices

- If you scored **20 - 30** your diet may be lacking important nutrients. Try to eat more balanced meals, with fresh ingredients.

- **Less than 20** your poor diet could be affecting your health. You need to improve your eating habits and you'll start to see the benefits quite quickly.

2. Fitness

Column	Count	Value	Score
A's		x 3	
B's		x 2	

Column	Count	Value	Score
C's		x 0	
-	-	**Total...**	

Assessment:

- If you scored **40 - 45** you're quite fit and in good shape
- If you have **30 - 39** you're probably not a couch potato, but you should look at increasing your activity level
- If you scored **20 - 30** you should be improving your fitness. Start with those areas where you scored '0'
- **Less than 20** you definitely need to start on a fitness routine - but check with your doctor first!

3. Stress Level

Column	Count	Value	Score
A's		x 3	
B's		x 2	
C's		x 0	
-	-	**Total...**	

Assessment:

- If you scored **over 40** you're really laid back! No worries regarding stress...
- If you scored between **30 and 39** you're a generally relaxed person and not too stressed.
- In the **15 to 30 range** you're experiencing a greater than normal level of stress, that will end up affecting your health. Try to follow some of the recommendations I suggest in the chapter on Stress.

- **Less than 15,** you are definitely stressed out. Read the chapter on Stress again for some helpful suggestions. If you're not exercising regularly, try to find the time to do this. You should also check with your doctor.

4. General Health

Column	Count	Value	Score
A's		x 3	
B's		x 2	
C's		x 0	
-	-	**Total...**	

Assessment:

- If you scored **38 - 42,** you look like you're enjoying reasonably good health (but see the caution above)
- In the **25 to 37 range** you're probably about average, depending on your age as well
- **18 - 24,** you're not in top shape and you should start on a wellness improvement program.
- **Less than 18,** the best place to start is with a visit to your doctor. Also check with a reliable nutritionist about your diet.

5. Brain Health

Column	Count	Value	Score
A's		x 3	
B's		x 2	
C's		x 0	
-	-	**Total...**	

Assessment:

- If you scored **16 - 21** your brain health looks good.
- In the **11 to 15** range you're still doing quite well.
- **7 - 10**, you should start following the recommendations in the Brain Health chapter
- **Less than 7** it looks like you're having problems. Definitely check with your doctor.

~~~~~~~~~~~~~~

Putting It All together

Now take your separate scores for each part of the test and enter them into the following table.

*Because the **Brain Health** part of the questionnaire contained a fewer number of questions, multiply your score from this section by two (see below).*

Section	Your Score
1. Nutrition	
2. Fitness	
3. Stress Level	
4. General Health	
5. Brain Health **x 2**	
Total Wellness Score	

Assessment

- If your total wellness score is **192 - 222:**
  Excellent, your score indicates a very high level of wellness. You don't need to make any drastic changes to your lifestyle. But please keep on reading the next chapters - we can all improve!
- If you scored between **133 and 191:**

Well done, this is an above average score, especially if you are 60 or older.

- If your score was **81 to 132:**

  This is an average score and you need to seriously consider making some life changes now if you don't want to end up like so many other people today who are aged 70 or over.

- **If you scored less than 81:**

  You definitely can and should improve your wellness level. I urge you to make some changes and start following the recommendations in the next couple of chapters.

Don't be discouraged if your score was lower than you'd hoped. The whole idea of the questionnaire is simply to give you an idea of where your wellness level is at today. Based on this you can start to consider the lifestyle changes you need to make to improve. If you do this, you should start to see some small improvements in your wellness level in as little as two or three weeks.

~~~~~~~~~~~~~~~~~~~~~

Making Positive Changes Become Habits

If you're serious about improving your lifestyle this is one of the most important chapters to read in the whole book. It shows how I started adopting some good habits and getting rid of some not-so-good ones! I'm including it to help you make the changes that lead to healthier choices. In my case, some things just fell into place, while for others I had to work really hard. As I've said before, it took me a long time to achieve the fairly healthy lifestyle I enjoy today - I'm sure you can do it faster.

Advice is easy to give and hard to take
I don't blame you if you're thinking it's easy for me to sit here and tell you all the things you should be doing, when I don't have a hectic life like yours to deal with every day.

But if you really do want to improve your current lifestyle so you can enjoy a much more rewarding and healthier retirement, then I urge you - don't wait too long to do something about it!

Like some folks I have known personally who:

- Nearly died from flu' complications, before deciding to quit drinking
- Suffered from a heart attack and after recovering, started a walking program
- Had a mild stroke, before changing his unhealthy diet, which included a smoked meat sandwich for lunch almost every day
- Had a triple-bypass, before cutting back on smoking

and I'm sure you've heard lots of similar stories...

About Habits
A habit is a regular behavior that tends to occur subconsciously. We don't have to think about it too much. Brushing your teeth every day, taking a shower when you

wake up, or relaxing with a drink after work are some simple examples.

All habits follow the same three-step process. First of all there's the cue that triggers the habit. For example you wake up in the morning and automatically head for the bathroom. Next is the routine, which is the actual activity itself. Finally, there is the reward, like feeling awake and refreshed when you step out of the shower. It's the reward part of the loop that reinforces the habit.

Your brain is not actively involved in the process. Driving to work is a good example, you get in the car, set off and then arrive at the office without thinking about the directions you needed to take to get there.

The fact that your brain is not too involved in the behavior is why we often end up with bad habits as well as good ones. If you consciously looked at the cigarette every time you took it out of the packet and then told yourself 'this is killing me' as you light up, you might be more inclined to quit

Knowing how habits are formed and how they work can be a big help when you are trying to make changes in your life.

The Cue is the Key
Now here's the important part - how do you transform the idea, or goal into a regular routine for achieving your objectives? It's easier than it seems - setting up a cue is the key to the whole habit-forming process.

Let's take a real example from my own experience, I was really wanting to do more strength training. This became something of a priority for me. My upper body was relatively weak compared to my legs and trunk.

We already had a Bowflex machine set up in the basement! But in spite of this I still could not get into doing the workouts on a regular basis. Usually I just forgot about it and did something else that I felt was pressing.

Then I got the idea of using a cue, or trigger, to get me going. This turned out to be extremely simple. I said to myself, "every day after I finish my coffee in the morning, I'll check to see if it's a weight-training day". If so I'd go to the basement and do 20 minutes of exercise on the Bowflex machine.

Well, it did take one or two times to get me going, but now, every day as I'm finishing my cup of coffee, I think about the strength training workout., which I do on alternate days. It's become a habit for me and I actually don't feel right if I have to skip the workout for some reason.

You may be thinking this is too simple, it won't work for me. But it can. Remember the habit process description above:

1. The Cue that triggers the habit
2. The Routine that you carry out
3. The Reward

The Cue isn't in first place for nothing. When I smoked I had lots of unconscious cues that would trigger my habit

- I'd get a phone call, start talking and light up a cigarette
- I'd have a coffee and reach for a cigarette
- After finishing a meal, I'd have a cigarette
- I'd have a beer after work and start smoking...

You see the pattern. Cues are a lot more powerful than we would think, because they occur at the subconscious level. I didn't have to say to myself "Hey, I'm having a coffee - I need a cigarette!" I just automatically reached for the packet.

If you can create cues for good habits you want to form then you're well on the way to achieving your goal. Let's try out an example with one of the goals we mention in the next chapter.

Creating Cues - a detailed example

The original goal to help stress reduction was:

> "*Start an aerobic exercise program*"

which becomes more detailed and better defined as:

> "*I'm going to do a slow run/walk combination for 30 minutes, three times a week at lunch times*"

Now let's assume you are going to do this from your workplace, where changing and shower facilities are available. The first think we need to do is get into the habit of taking some workout gear with us to work. Here's a possible cue:

> "*As I finish my morning coffee, I'll pack my gym bag*"

or

> "*when I reach for my briefcase I'll remember to grab my gym bag as well*".

This should become routine after a short while. Now once we're at work it's a whole different ball game. Lots of different things can come up to throw us off schedule. So the first thing you can do is schedule the workout for three days of the week. However we need a fallback because quite often you may not be able to make the time.

So we need a fallback cue. This is very simple - use the word "*lunch*" so if someone asks you what you're doing at lunch time, you are going to think "*is this a workout day for me*"? Or, you might start getting hungry and thinking of "*lunch*" - this should also act as the trigger to check if it's a workout day.

Now all this might seem like an incredibly detailed process to go through just to get started on an exercise program. In fact it may well be! Nevertheless, it's worth going through the mental exercise at least. There's lots of opportunities that will come up, while you're trying to break bad habits or form better ones, when you'll need to use a similar cue creation technique.

When does a new behavior become a habit?

If you ask Google this question, you'll often get the answer - "it depends!". You'll also find '66 days' as another frequently quoted response. Don't be discouraged - I've found you can often change a routine in 1-2 weeks. I'm hoping you will be able to get your new lifestyle changes firmly entrenched in your daily routine before too long. That's why it's so important to:

- Keep your goals short, simple and above all, do-able
- Take it in easy steps
- Make sure the Reward part of the new habit gets emphasized, either a mental pat on the back, or as something more physical like losing weight, or both!
- Keep motivated

Once you've achieved a healthier lifestyle, believe me, you won't want to go back, because you'll be feeling so much better and more energetic than before.

~ ~ ~ ~ ~ ~ ~ ~ ~ ~ ~ ~ ~ ~ ~ ~ ~ ~ ~ ~

Getting (and Staying) Healthy

OK - this is where the rubber hits the road, so to speak. If you've completed the Wellness Self Assessment in the previous chapter you should know what your weak points are. The major challenge you are facing is how do you make <u>lasting</u> changes in your lifestyle that will improve your wellness. So many people start out with the best of intentions, but then gradually slip back into their old ways.

I think you can be different - don't be like those others.

This chapter outlines some of the steps you can take right away to start getting healthier and feeling better. Remember though, this book can't motivate you to modify your lifestyle and adopt some healthy changes. <u>You have to motivate yourself to do this.</u> Hopefully what you've been reading will act as the motivational trigger you need to convince yourself that you need to start making changes <u>now</u> - not tomorrow, not next week nor January 1st... Why not re-read the chapters on Motivation and Habit-forming now, before you continue?

The way to get healthier sounds very simple and self-evident:

1. Gradually remove the things from your life that are negatively affecting your wellness
2. Gradually introduce the things that will improve your wellness

I've added the word 'Gradually' to these steps because very few of us are capable of making major permanent changes in our behavior that quickly. Still, we can all encounter problems when it comes to actually accomplishing these two straightforward goals, even if we're motivated to do so. I believe the answer lies in our ability, or rather our inability, to change existing habits and create new and better ones. For this reason I devoted the previous chapter to the topic of forming new habits and getting rid of bad ones.

In the meantime it helps to look at some of the positive gains I made from being able to change my lifestyle. You can expect the same benefits if you can change your life and improve your wellness. Here are just a few:

- A stronger immune system
- Fewer common illnesses, like colds and 'flu
- Reduced risks of chronic disease
- More vitality
- A positive outlook on life
- Slowing down the effects of aging
- Enjoying your retirement years

Here's the question - what do you need to start doing today to achieve this?

In my case I didn't have a plan to start with and just gradually improved my lifestyle over time. It would have been better though if I'd had some definite goals. Here's my advice for getting started.

- Make being healthier a priority in your life. This is always hard to do if you are not actually sick, but this is your first goal.

- Take an interest in all things related to healthy living; - buy a magazine, watch TV programs like The Doctors and Dr. Oz (although don't believe everything you see). Netflix has some acclaimed documentaries on nutrition. You can also do some Internet research on health or exercise topics you're interested in (again, with the Internet its a case of 'read with care' and double check what you think you've learned).

- Don't try to make any immediate drastic changes in your diet or exercise right away, you could easily get discouraged and give up on the whole idea. Change things gradually.

- Set some goals you know you can reach, such as reducing your sugar intake, or losing five pounds if you need to, or eating less fast food. Don't expect a miracle, you can't undo twenty years of less-than-healthy living in two weeks or even two months. You should start to see some improvements early on though.

Don't wait until you're sick to start getting healthy!

♥ *Health Hint*

If you are going to change your current lifestyle you should schedule a visit with your doctor. Get a physical check-up and tell him of any dietary changes you plan on making. If you are seriously out of shape, ask him/her for his/her advice on how much exercise you can safely undertake.

I went to see my doctor when I turned forty and it was the first time I'd been in years. As it turned out youth was on my side and even though I had recently been a regular smoker I was good to go.

Recruit Friends

The hardest part about making changes in your life is actually sticking with the plan. It helps if you can get involved with other people who have similar goals and interests. For example a few of my friends in the local running club decided they wanted to lose some weight after the Christmas holidays. They organized a little contest over a three month period to see who could slim down the most. They all lost weight and the winner dropped 20 lbs.!

If you have any friends who are also interested in getting healthier you could talk to them and try to get your own wellness group going. As they say, there's strength in numbers and the friendly competition and mutual encouragement helps a lot.

Decide What You Want

If you completed the Wellness Questionnaire you should know which areas of your lifestyle need work. It helps to write these down. For example;

- I'm eating too much red meat
- I'm not sleeping as well as I should
- I'm not very fit
- I'm eating out too often
- I worry too much

Don't worry if you end up with a huge list, you won't be working on everything all at once!

Prioritize

Look down the list and try to pick out the top five or so, based on these criteria

1. Can I start on this right away?
2. Do I have the time to do it?
3. Is it a major priority for me?

Now to be able to fit in extra activities like walking or cooking healthier meals, you'll need to re-arrange your current schedule. You might decide you'll have to get up earlier in the morning and this then becomes one of your top goals.

Create Attainable Sub-goals

If you try to do everything at once you'll probably end up getting discouraged and may give up on the idea altogether. It's much easier and more rewarding if you create mini-goals - think of them as steps - that make up the main goal.

When I enter a full marathon event and I'm standing at the start line, I don't focus on the finish line 26 miles away. It's too far away and the mileage count would go by very slowly. Instead I think about my first goal of 10K or 6 miles. When I reach that point I do a self check on how I'm feeling - should I slow down, speed up or continue at the same pace? I also look ahead to my next checkpoint at 10 miles. Breaking up a long race into manageable smaller chunks makes it easier on both the mind and the body.

You can do the same with your wellness goals and initially pick ones that are easily achievable. You could have an exercise goal that says ' I'll start a walking program this week'. Once you've started you could add 'I'll walk a minimum of two miles on each walk, three times a week'. You can then build on your achievements as you go along.

Let's say your goal is to reduce your stress level, which you think you can do in several ways:

- start an aerobic exercise program
- do some meditation
- leave for work a half hour earlier and avoid the heavy traffic

These then become your sub-goals for reaching the main goal of reducing your stress levels.

Quantify Your Goals

Let's take the 'Eating less red meat' goal as an example. If you said to yourself 'I'm going to eat less red meat' this is not going to mean much in real life terms. To your brain it's not very clear - 'less' is not a number and there is no schedule. When will you eat less red meat, exactly?

So, try to re-frame your goal something like this:

> *'I'll eat red meat a maximum of twice a week for the next month'.*

Another example from the fitness category could be:

> *'I'm going to do a slow run/walk combination for 30 minutes, three times a week at lunch times'*

instead of the original 'start an aerobic exercise program'

You see how precisely defined these goals are? Not only that, they are also very achievable. You're not taking on too much at once.

Of course a strong desire for change has got to be there if you really want to improve your lifestyle. I find it helps to focus on the end goal - being fit and healthy into your seventies so you can enjoy life. Take a look around at the state of health of many people already in this age group - if that doesn't convince you to start making changes, nothing will.

You just need to believe that a healthier lifestyle really will reduce your risks of age-related problems.

> *It's like saving for retirement, the earlier you start the more you'll have in the health bank later on in life.*

Healthy Habits

If you can persevere you'll find that in a reasonably short timeframe, you'll start to adopt some healthier habits. Here's a few of mine that I've adopted over time:

- I rarely buy a food item without scrutinizing the label. (By the way, I hate those jokers who print an almost unreadable ingredients list on the label using a tiny black font on a red background - who are they trying to kid? I just give up and move on to an alternate product)
- I maintain a keen interest on anything I come across related to health and wellness. I'm not always convinced but I keep an open mind on some of the so-called alternative cures that you see reported quite often on the Internet and in the media.

- Added sugar and sweeteners in food are really bad, so I've cut way back on these.
- I eat red meats (like beef, pork, or lamb) less than three times per week and try to include one or two days when I eat only vegetarian meals.
- I do 10 minutes of mild stretching every morning as soon as I get up which helps a lot to ease the usual aches and pains we experience at that time of day.
- I get outside (unless the weather is really bad!) for an hour or more of exercise almost every day of the year.
- I try to do some strength training workouts three times a week.

These are just some examples of my own lifestyle habits - I'm not suggesting you do exactly the same things. But the above are now part of my daily and weekly routine. I don't feel good if I can't include them on a regular basis. On the other hand, I'm not overly concerned if I deviate from them occasionally.

Nutrition

This is usually one area where people can start to make improvements right away, like today! Chances are, if you are working every day and you are like I used to be, then you eat out a lot, eat processed foods and do very little food preparation from scratch. I now know this is not the road to long-term health.

Consistently eating the wrong foods has a very detrimental effect on us, as it...

- weakens our immune system
- upsets our digestive tract
- decreases brain acuity

Yes, food is that powerful. I've always believed the old saying "You are what you eat" - I just never realized to what extent this was true. Nowadays study after study has validated this statement.

Juicing

Buy a juicing machine. We have two at home - a traditional juicer that separates the pulp from the juice and a Nutri-bullet that operates more like a powerful blender. I like the latter because there's no waste and cleanup is a breeze. However the juice you get from the regular juicing machine is much more concentrated.

Why is juicing so important? It allows us to increase our intake of very healthy vegetables, including kale, spinach and broccoli as well as fruits like blueberries and kiwi. My wife and I often make a juice for lunch, accompanied by a dip like hummus or black bean.

More Nutrition Tips

In the section on nutrition, I talked about good foods you should be eating and not-so-good ones you should be avoiding or at least cutting back. Depending on your present diet I don't expect you can make the switch overnight - it took me long enough. What you can do right away though is to look at what you eat frequently and start cutting back on things that are definitely in the not-good category. Some of these would be:

Sugar-loaded Foods like pastries, donuts, sodas, candies and some breakfast cereals. The FDA recommends we consume less than 40 grams of added sugar per day. That's equivalent to a small can of soda, or 10 regular size sugar cubes!

Processed Meats like pepperoni, bacon, salami, hot dogs etc. The World Health Organization recent put this food category into Group 1 - Carcinogenic to Humans. Eating just 50g (less than 2 ounces) of processed meat per day can increase your risk of cancer by 18%, so I don't eat very much of this type of food.

Hydrogenated Fats or trans fats are found in deep-fried foods, fast food, some margarine products, many baked goods and packaged snacks and more.

You might be saying "Hey - I like a lot of this stuff, how am I going to cut it out of my diet?" Well it's kind of like quitting smoking, some people can quit cold turkey while others reduce gradually. I suggest you just try cutting back on the above foods.

Substitutes

Another thing we've done is to substitute some of the above foods with healthier choices:

Honey - use this instead of simple table sugar. While honey is essentially the same as sugar, it's much more complex and takes longer to breakdown in your body, reducing the spike you get from the same amount of ordinary sugar. Honey also contains trace nutrients that are good for you.

Bagels - if you like donuts and pastries for breakfast, try switching to whole grain bagels with cream cheese. This may not be the healthiest food, but it's way better for you than a sugar donut.

Dark Chocolate - if you like chocolates and other candies, give dark chocolate a try instead. It is much better for you and has proven health benefits. It contains half the amount of sugar or less, than regular chocolate. The amount of sugar decreases the higher the amount of cacao present; the 85% cacao version has only 16 grams of sugar in a 100 gram bar compared to 50 grams for milk chocolate.

Baked Potato Chips - these are somewhat better for you than the regular deep fried variety. However I've tried them and find they're not as tasty. The Kettle brand of chips, although fried, is a healthier choice than many other brands and I like the taste.

Popcorn - never mind the chips, try this snack instead. It has lots of nutritive value, is low in calories and is full of anti-oxidants. However, the popular microwaveable kind is not so good and usually contains chemical additives, like the diacetyl used to give it a buttery taste. To make things worse the popcorn bags themselves are lined with chemical products - chips would be a better option in this case! To get all the benefits from popcorn, pop your own at home using organic corn if you can get it.

Butter - due to its high saturated fat content it seems weird proposing butter as a substitute for anything. However nutritional science now views butter as being not so bad for us after all. It is a natural product, especially butter from grass-fed dairy cows, compared to margarine and has none of the trans fats. You can also use a little butter or coconut butter as a healthier choice instead of vegetable oils for cooking.

The above is just a small list of foods you can start substituting for the less healthy ones. I'm sure you can find others that you'll really like.

How Much Food Do You Need?

Generally speaking we eat to much. According to U.S. government guidelines

> *"Estimates range from 1,600 to 2,400 calories per day for adult women and 2,000 to 3,000 calories per day for adult men. Within each category, the low end of the range is for sedentary individuals; the high end of the range is for active individuals. Calorie needs generally decrease for adults as they age."*

(Source:
health.gov/dietaryguidelines/2015/guidelines/appendix-2/)

Obviously the more physically active you are the more energy from food you'll need. However many people with desk jobs are eating more than the recommended amount for an active person or an athlete. The average American consumes over 3,500 calories per day!

So try to exercise some portion control and keep an eye on the total calories you are taking in every day.

Exercise

Another thing you can start on is to include some regular exercise time in your schedule. If you can focus on just being more active this will help. In an earlier chapter I came up with a few ideas like climbing stairs at work instead of always using the elevator, parking your car further from the store when you are shopping and not sitting for more than 30 minutes at any one time. Several studies have shown that:

The less you sit, the longer you'll live

But to reap some serious health benefits, you need to get going on a regular exercise program. Why not review the section 'Keeping Fit' right now to refresh your memory on some of the suggestions and pointers about exercising.

The biggest challenge facing many of us who want to get fitter is trying to find the time for regular workouts in our busy schedules. A first step is to make it a priority right up there with all the others in your life! If you don't do this and just try to fit it in whenever you can, then it probably won't work.

I know this because I tried it myself and my whole getting fitter plan became very hit and miss. I didn't really get anywhere until I joined the Lunch Time Fitness club at my local YMCA. Then things really improved for me, I was able to do several different workouts during the week, with a friendly group of people who were always handy with advice if I needed it.

Some people may say they're in a high-power, high-stress job like a lawyer or a doctor and just can't take the time to follow an exercise program. People in stressful jobs actually need exercise more than the average person. It comes down to a choice between finding the time or suffering from declining health. I see people running past my window at 6:30AM and I know they are motivated to keeping fit.

If you're already doing some kind of workout it's a lot easier to build on this than if you're starting from scratch. But if you're just getting going in a fitness program, start slow and build up - you don't want to do much at first anyway. The secret is to simply develop a do-able routine that you can fit into your day on a regular basis.

Reduce Stress

This is something most of in modern society need to do and it's quite complementary to our other wellness goals. However in some ways it's one of the hardest to achieve. Mental relaxation is not a big part of our culture and it's not something we grow up with. Yoga classes can help but they take time. Exercise helps a lot, especially aerobic exercise like cycling or running. Good nutrition also plays a part in keep your stress down.

If you feel that you are more stressed than you should be, re-read the section on the power of the mind and see if there's something, however small, that you can start doing today to reduce your stress level. Remember that stress is a root cause of many illnesses. Even though you think you are handling it fine today, you are unknowingly opening the door to many chronic health issues. These may not show up right away - it may take two years, it may take ten. But the odds are your overall level of wellness will be affected.

Summary

So to summarize the steps you can take to start getting healthy:

1. You'll work on replacing unhealthy habits with healthier ones
2. You'll make 'improving your wellness' a priority in your life
3. You'll check in with your doctor and other health professionals
4. You'll try to team up with others who have similar objectives
5. You'll set some health goals you can achieve fairly quickly
6. You'll improve on the kinds of food you eat
7. You'll start to reduce the amount of sugar, salt, fat and processed foods in your diet
8. You'll begin a regular exercise program
9. You'll try to lower your stress level
10. You'll stay motivated to stick with the plan!

Theses are all things that I did, over a number of years...

Staying Healthy

Getting started is the hardest part - once you get going you'll have some momentum to help you to the next level. Perhaps you will have made some new friends if you joined a club or a gym. Maybe family members are involved in trying to improve their health. Either way, it all helps to keep you motivated and keep on going. The biggest impact will come just from the way you feel. You'll be more alert, you'll have more energy, you might have dropped a few pounds and you'll have a more positive outlook on life.

One of the advantages of creating healthy habits I found is that you don't have to stick rigorously to your diet or your exercise programs all the time. You can take a few days off if you feel like it - chances are, you'll miss the healthy alternatives you've gotten used to.

So what would make you lapse back into your old ways? Unfortunately there are quite a few reasons why this can happen - I know because it's happened to me. It doesn't hurt to think in advance about things that could have a negative effect on you. Ask yourself what "would I do if..." or "how would I handle this", then if the worst does happen you won't be totally unprepared.

1. Injuries
If you've taken up a new sport and then suffer an injury that may take several weeks to heal, you could abandon the sport altogether along with your other wellness goals. I've seen this happen to people I know.

2. Life Changes
Life is full of unexpected twists and turns. You may get a new job with new responsibilities and feel you don't have as much time to devote to your wellness activities. Maybe your job requires a lot of travel, which is always a problem when you're try to maintain a healthy lifestyle.

3. Sickness
In spite of your efforts you may get sick from anything such as the 'flu to something more serious. This will definitely interrupt your routine and you'll need to make a special effort to get back on track as you recover. Now the good thing about improving your wellness is, as time goes by, you'll have a much stronger immune system. You'll be able to fight off a lot of common sickness threats and shorten your recovery time if you do fall ill.

4. Relationships
Relationships can be stressful at any time. A change in your relationship, such as divorce, can be really

upsetting both emotionally and physically. This is the time when you really need to hang in and keep up with your wellness program - it will help you get through this difficult period.

The above are just a few examples of the many life-changing events that can throw you off your intended health and fitness track. A lot depends on how deeply ingrained your new habits were. If you're just getting started on building a healthier lifestyle, it's easier to get discouraged and return to your old habits. In this case you may have to remind yourself why you wanted to improve your wellness in the first place. It's because you don't want to end up like the vast majority of elderly people who are unable to enjoy their older years due to failing health.

I hope this chapter will help you come up with your own plan for getting and staying healthy. You'll have to work at it and keep it up, but the results will be long-lasting and definitely worthwhile.

~ ~

A Wellness Improvement Program

Self Assessment Results

How well did you score in the five main areas of the wellness self-assessment?

- Nutrition
- Fitness
- Stress Level
- General Health
- Brain Health

This chapter is organized according to your overall wellness score and your score in each section. I must emphasize however that everyone of us is different and you must use your own judgment when it comes to making choices and decisions about lifestyle changes.

There are some things I recommend you do, whatever your score on the Wellness questionnaire. As I mentioned in the last chapter:

- Plan to get check-ups with your health professionals - doctor, dentist and optician as needed.
- Make sure you're really committed to improving your wellness and are prepared to make the necessary lifestyle changes.
- Try and get a friend or friends with similar goals involved with you. Join an appropriate club or a class - it helps keep you motivated.

Goals

Try and set some simple goals for yourself that you can achieve within a month. It always helps to write them down. You can have longer term goals too, but you're going to focus on the immediate ones. Here's a few examples:

- "Starting this week, I'll eat cold water fish for dinner twice a week, every week"
- "Starting today, I'll drink tea instead of my usual afternoon coffee"
- "To help reduce my sugar intake I'll check the (added) sugar content on every processed food product I purchase"

How To Follow The Program

Check your total score for the Wellness Questionnaire and read the recommendations for the level indicated by your score, as follows:

- Level 1 - if you scored 80 or less
- Level 2 - 81 to 132
- Level 3 - 133 to 191
- Level 4 - 192 to 222

Each level contains some suggestions you can use to improve in the wellness areas covered in the questionnaire, Nutrition, Fitness, Stress, General health and Brain health.

Imagine you had a total wellness score of 121. This falls in the level 2 range, so you would go to this section of the plan. then look back at the score you obtained for each category.

Level 1	OK, let's get started on improving your wellness level! You probably scored low on most of the categories, but don't be discouraged.
	Focus on Nutrition, Fitness and General Health to start with. If you scored low on the Health category then a consultation with your physician is definitely needed.
	If you're a smoker, you need to do everything you can to try to quit. It's affecting your fitness right now and will impact your health as you age.
	If you are working at a desk and are sitting a lot, try to be more active. Even taking a five minute break every half hour and walking around will help.

Level 2	You're in the average range, so there's definitely room to improve. Many people score in this group because of their dietary habits, so review your daily food intake and try to follow some of the recommendations outlined in the plan below.
	If you scored high in the Stress category, remember that regular exercise can help a lot to reduce chronic stress. Increasing you level of activity is very important, so try and make this a priority. Start a regular exercise program by joining a gym or a club, but you need to take it easy to start with and build up slowly.
Level 3	Your wellness level is above average! Typically at this level you are doing a lot of the right things to maintain a good level of wellness. You can probably make some nutrition improvements, like eating more fish (except for vegetarians) and increasing your omega-3 intake. See below for more details. Stress level is another area where many people can make improvements.
Level 4	Looks like you're in really good shape. You just need to keep on the same path and maybe try to improve on areas where you scored low.

The table below guides you through the different parts of the Wellness test, with suggestions for you to follow, depending on your score in each segment.

Detailed Wellness Improvement Plan

Your score ...	---- 1 ---- 30 or less	---- 2 ---- 30 - 39	---- 3 ---- 40 - 45
Nutrition	- Eat more fresh fruit daily - Try to get 3 servings of vegetables each day - Meat eaters - eat cold water fish at least twice per week - Take a good quality fish oil supplement	-Follow the recommendations in column 1. - Make sure to eat plenty of spinach, kale and broccoli - Eat more plant-based dinners every week, without meat or fish	- You are eating quite a healthy diet. Review your answers to the Nutrition questions and make any needed changes.

Your score ...	---- 1 ---- 30 or less	---- 2 ---- 30 - 39	---- 3 ---- 40 - 45
	- Reduce your intake of sweet foods and sugar		
Fitness	- Start a moderate exercise program such as walking - Do some strength training, starting with very light weights - Do some stretching to improve your flexibility	- Join a gym or club and start a regular workout program - Be generally more active on a daily basis - climb stairs, walk more - Set some fitness goals that you want to reach within the next six months	- You're doing well with this score. Remember though - 'train don't strain' If you sit a lot all day, take a standing break every 30 minutes or so.
Stress Level	- Re-read the chapters on Stress and Sleep - Identify the main reasons you are stressed. Next, work out ways you can try to reduce your stress level	- It takes time and practice to de-stress. Try exercise and meditation - Unplug! Turn off all the gadgets, phone, TV, and go for a long walk. You'll feel great at the end of the day	- Even the most laid-back folks can get stressed. Just realize when it's happening and take steps to counteract it.
General health	- If you smoke, try your best to quit - Reduce your stress level - Try to start a light exercise program - Discuss your wellness goals with your doctor	- See the suggestions in column 1 - Start to improve your exercise level	- You're in good shape, just continue to get regular check-ups.
Brain health	- Use the 'Brain Age' test as a guide to what you need to do here - Exercise your brain - do some crosswords, puzzles, etc. every day	- As you age it's always beneficial to follow the suggestions in column 1	- Keep on exercising the brain! Follow the suggestions in column 1

Timetable

Months 1 - 2

Follow the suggestions above according to how you scored. Don't try to do everything at once - focus on the things that need it most.

At the end of month 2, re-take the test. Did you improve? If so follow the recommendations for the next score over in the table. Otherwise, review what you need to do and keep on trying!

Months 3 - 4

You should be feeling better and more energetic. At the end of month four take the Wellness test again and move along in the table score as appropriate.

Months 5 - 8

You're well into the program at this point and should be feeling the difference. A lot of the positive changes you've made should have become regular habits by now.

Months 9 - 12

One year later! Congratulations if you've stuck with the program. If you get another physical exam, your doctor should also notice the difference. Remember to re-do the Wellness test every year, just to make sure you are keeping on track.

~~~~~~~~~~~~~~~~~~~~~

A Typical Day

Many of us cringe at the thought of trying to follow a healthy life style - having to exercise regularly and avoiding many of the foods we like. I want to show you that it's not as hard as you think, by describing a typical day out of my life.

Since many of the readers will still be leading busy working lives, I've gone back a few years to when I was employed as a project manager on a large computer project for an insurance company based in the Midwest.

5:30 - 6:00 AM
Yes, we're early risers in this part of the country! First of all I do about 10 minutes of stretching and warm-up exercises. Next I have my daily 'start-up' drink, consisting of:

- hot water
- a little fresh lemon juice
- a tablespoon of apple cider vinegar
- 1/2 teaspoon of unfiltered honey

This is a good cleansing drink and a great way to start your day. I really look forward to it and am disappointed if I can't have one for some reason.

Next it's bathroom duties...

After a shower and a shave I'm ready for breakfast. Typically 1/2 slice of toast with cheese and 1/2 slice with peanut butter. Or a boiled egg instead of the cheese. I have a cup of coffee with the meal. After this I take a few vitamin supplements, C, CoQ10, Saw Palmetto, B complex.

Then it's a 15 minute drive to work, or on several days of the week I bike in which takes me about 40 minutes.

7:00 - 7:30AM
Now it's work time. Like most people today, I have a desk job. However there are lots of (too many!) meetings during the day, so I do get to walk from one building to another. I also make a point of getting up from my desk every 30 minutes or so. During this time I'll walk around and maybe visit with members of my project team. A couple of them are at stand-up work-stations, a recent innovation in the company. Around 9:30 I usually take a coffee break and either get a bran muffin, or have a delicious health cookie that my wife makes.

At lunch I eat at the cafeteria about 11:30 and today I have a salad. They have a great salad bar that's better than most restaurants I've been in. I make sure to add beans and chickpeas to my selection, as well as things like beets and broccoli. Trust me - it tastes much better than it sounds! After lunch, if I didn't bike in and I have no meetings scheduled, I take a one mile walk around the company complex.

Then it's back to work. Since I began eating healthier and having lighter lunches I don't get that tired feeling I used to get in the mid-afternoon. I try to quit around 4PM, but that's not always possible... The company has a flex hours schedule and if it's Friday I leave at lunch time for the weekend. This is often one of my biking days.

4:30PM
When I get home my wife and I may go for a walk, or a run. I'm trying to run about 4 times a week. Instead of a run I sometimes do about half an hour of strength training (about three times a week). After that we might relax with a cold beer! Yes I do drink alcohol, but I try to average two drinks a day.

Then it's time for supper, we eat a healthy meal on most days, but sometimes we do 'cheat' a little! Tonight I'm doing some salmon on the BBQ. I never use aluminum foil, I just put the salmon directly on the grill (which I sprayed with coconut oil) and move it frequently to avoid sticking. It tastes great! My wife always make some tasty dishes to go with the fish. We're having steamed asparagus and boiled red potatoes garnished with some herbs and spices.

7:30PM
After supper we often watch some TV and them I try to get to bed between 9:30 and 10PM. I do some word or logic puzzles to give the brain some exercise and then I'll often read a few pages of my current book (usually suspense fiction from authors like Steve Berry or David Baldacci).

I try to get to sleep by 10:30 because 5:30 seems to come around really quickly! I normally get a good night's sleep, maybe getting up once for a bathroom break. Then it's the next day - I usually wake up at the right time, but always have an alarm as back-up.

So that's it, I'm so used to doing things like the morning stretches or going for a workout that it's ingrained and I don't have to consciously force myself. Although, if I'm going for a run it's sometimes harder to get out of the door and start the workout when the weather is bad.

I realize you may have a totally different routine, but the key to improving your wellness is to make sure you're eating the right foods, avoiding the bad ones and doing some exercise. Taking some time to relax during the day also helps with the stress level. When I lived in Toronto I used to take public transport to work and found it way less stressful than driving.

~~~~~~~~~~~~~~~~~~~~~

My Top Ten Wellness Tips

As you've been reading this book you've probably noticed some topics I talk about often. I'd like to complete the book with a list of lifestyle tips - I've summarized below the ones I believe contribute a lot to a healthy life.

1. **Eat Your Veggies!**
   Dark leafy greens like spinach and kale, cruciferous vegetables like broccoli and cauliflower are chock full of healthful nutrients   I eat at least one serving of these every day. Salads are a great way to get enough of these beneficial foods.

2. **Get A Juicer**
   I swear by these and we try to have a juice from a veggie-fruit mix at least two or three times a week. It's a good way to get a concentrated amount of easily digestible nutrients into your body. (See 'Healthy Habits' in the Getting & Staying Healthy chapter)

3. **Eat More Fish**
   Most of us can benefit by adding more (preferably cold water) fish to our diet. The omega-3 essential fatty acid they contain is really healthy. We're also trying to redress the ratio of omega-6 to omega-3 in our bodies to about three to one, since Western diets are heavy in omega-6.
   I try to eat fresh fish when it's available, but so much fish these days is farm-raised. I'm not convinced that it's such a healthy choice as it used to be.

4. **Essential nutrients**
   Many of us are deficient in some important nutrients like magnesium, potassium and vitamin D. Review the chapter on this topic to make sure you are getting enough of the right foods, or take a supplement if not.

However I much prefer to get these essential nutrients from a natural food source, rather than a supplement.

5. **Early Morning Stretches**

Do your muscles feel a little stiff and achy when you get out of bed early in the morning? I know mine do. So I do this stretching routine I've been doing faithfully most days for twenty years. I first came across it in a book I read many years ago (unfortunately I don't remember the name). Anyway, it's a great way to limber up before you do anything else. See Appendix F for a description of these exercises.

However there's plenty of morning workout routines out there so just find one that you like and get into the habit of doing it every morning.

6. **Be Active**

Make getting out for some regular exercise a top priority in your life. There's so many long-term health benefits associated with doing this which you shouldn't ignore or put off doing until 'later' (remember that old saying "*later never comes*"!). Starting a regular exercise program was the thing that got me motivated to start improving my lifestyle as a whole.

If you can increase your overall activity level, by sitting less, walking more, climbing stairs and so on, that's even better.

7. **Visit Your Doctor**

Don't wait until you're sick - schedule a check up. Even if you are relatively young and in your forties it's a good idea to do this. Why? It gives you a benchmark of your physical condition that you can use for comparison as the years go by. This includes measures of your cholesterol levels, blood sugar etc. It may even identify some health issues you were completely unaware of.

8. Exercise Your Brain

You might think you're doing that every day when you go to work. And you are, to a limited extent. But you're actually doing the same kind of thing every day and your brain is only working within a set of parameters defined by the type of job you do. You need to expand the scope, so it's a good idea to get into the habit of doing crosswords, brain teasers, or even card games. The more you can mix it up the better off you'll be.

9. Think About Your Stress Level

That may sound a little weird, but we often just accept stress as a normal part of our lives. This is dangerous to your long-term health. Accepting the situation does not resolve it and you are actually living with a chronic stress condition that constantly works away at the foundation of your wellness. By thinking about it, you're taking the first step to fixing it!

Try to work some quiet, meditative time into your day. I read an article recently where the author described how he would meditate at odd times throughout the day, like waiting for his computer to boot up. I thought that was rather neat - why get all impatient watching a little wheel on your screen go round and round, when you can close your eyes and really relax?

10. Early to Bed

Sleep is really important to your overall well-being, especially as you start to get older. Unfortunately we usually keep on doing what we've done since we were younger and stay up until midnight. Then it's up again at 6:00 the next morning!

If you're in your late forties or over, try going to bed a little earlier each time, until you're at the point where you can count on 7 - 8 hours of restful sleep every night. Exercising regularly helps, because you'll be more tired out physically by the end of the day.

Conclusion

So that's it! I hope my story and advice will help you achieve your health goals. Based on my own experience I'm convinced that if you can adopt a healthier lifestyle then you will benefit greatly later on in your life.

On another note it's taken me quite a while to get my book to the published stage. I got side-tracked trying to find a conventional print publisher for 'Forty plus Thirty'. I was unsuccessful mainly because I was a complete unknown as far as the general public goes. So I turned to Amazon Kindle Publishing and so far it's working out really well. Thank you by the way for purchasing a copy of my book and I hope you can recommend it to your friends, and perhaps write a review on Kindle.

If you want to read lots of interesting articles about the many different aspects of wellness mentioned in this book, you can visit the 'Forty plus Thirty' website

http://www.fortyplusthirty.com/

Click on the References link to get easy access to the ninety+ main references I included as part of my research.

And finally:-
Just do it!

APPENDICES

APPENDIX A - Body Mass Index (BMI) Table

APPENDIX B - Natural Sources Of Key Essential Nutrients

APPENDIX C - Healthy Recipe Ideas

APPENDIX D - Facts On Fats and Oils

APPENDIX E - Morning Stretches

APPENDIX A - Body Mass Index (BMI)

(See a Metric version on the next page)

To find your BMI value, simply look up your height in feet and inches in the left hand column and then read across until you find the column closest to your weight. Your BMI is at the top and bottom of that column

BMI >>	20	22	24	26	28	30	32	34	36	38	40	44	48	50
Height	-------			Body Weight In pounds							-------			
4' 10"	96	105	115	124	134	143	153	162	172	181	191	210	229	239
4' 11"	99	109	119	128	138	148	158	168	178	188	198	217	237	247
5' 0"	102	112	123	133	143	153	163	174	184	194	204	225	245	255
5' 1"	106	116	127	137	148	158	169	180	190	201	211	232	254	264
5' 2"	109	120	131	142	153	164	175	186	196	207	218	240	262	273
5' 3"	113	124	135	146	158	169	180	191	203	214	225	248	270	282
5' 4"	116	128	140	151	163	174	186	197	209	221	232	256	279	291
5' 5"	120	132	144	156	168	180	192	204	216	228	240	264	288	300
5' 6"	124	136	148	161	173	186	198	210	223	235	247	272	297	309
5' 7"	127	140	153	166	178	191	204	217	230	242	255	280	306	319
5' 8"	131	144	158	171	184	197	210	223	236	249	262	289	315	328
5' 9"	135	149	162	176	189	203	216	230	243	257	270	297	324	338
5' 10"	139	153	167	181	195	209	222	236	250	264	278	306	334	348
5' 11"	143	157	172	186	200	215	229	243	257	272	286	315	343	358
6' 0"	147	162	177	191	206	221	235	250	265	279	294	324	353	368
6' 1"	151	166	182	197	212	227	242	257	272	288	302	333	363	378
6' 2"	155	171	186	202	218	233	249	264	280	295	311	342	373	389
6' 3"	160	176	192	208	224	240	256	272	287	303	319	351	383	399
6' 4"	164	180	197	213	230	246	263	279	295	312	328	361	394	410
BMI	20	22	24	26	28	30	32	34	36	38	40	44	48	50

Here's what the BMI values mean:
- 18.00 - 24.9   Normal

- 25.00 - 29.9   Overweight
- 30.00 - 39.9   Obese
- Over 40.00   Severe obesity

Body Mass Index (BMI) Table - Metric Version

To find your BMI value, simply look up your height in centimetres in the left hand column and then read across until you find the column closest to your weight in kilograms. Your BMI is at the top of that column

BMI >>	20	22	24	26	28	30	32	34	36	38	40	44	48	50
Height	-------				Body Weight In Kilograms							------		
147	44	48	52	56	61	65	69	73	78	82	87	95	104	108
150	45	49	54	58	63	67	72	76	81	85	90	98	108	112
152	46	51	56	60	65	69	74	79	83	88	93	102	111	116
155	48	53	58	62	67	72	77	82	86	91	96	105	115	120
157	49	54	59	64	69	74	79	84	89	94	99	109	119	124
160	51	56	61	66	72	77	82	87	92	97	102	112	122	128
163	53	58	64	68	74	79	84	89	95	100	105	116	127	132
165	54	60	65	71	76	82	87	93	98	103	109	120	131	136
168	56	62	67	73	78	84	90	95	101	107	112	123	135	140
170	58	64	69	75	81	87	93	98	104	110	116	127	139	145
173	59	65	72	78	83	89	95	101	107	113	119	131	143	149
175	61	68	73	80	86	92	98	104	110	117	122	135	147	153
178	63	69	76	82	88	95	101	107	113	120	126	139	151	158
180	65	71	78	84	91	98	104	110	117	123	130	143	156	162
183	67	73	80	87	93	100	107	113	120	127	133	147	160	167
185	68	75	83	89	96	103	110	117	123	131	137	151	165	171
188	70	78	84	92	99	106	113	120	127	134	141	155	169	176
191	73	80	87	94	102	109	116	123	130	137	145	159	174	181
193	74	82	89	97	104	112	119	127	134	142	149	164	179	186
BMI	20	22	24	26	28	30	32	34	36	38	40	44	48	50

Here's what the BMI values mean:

- 18.00 - 24.9   Normal

- 25.00 - 29.9   Overweight
- 30.00 - 39.9   Obese
- Over 40.00   Severe obesity

APPENDIX B - Natural Sources Of Key Essential Nutrients

The DV refers to the Daily Value - the recommended amount needed on a daily basis

1. Magnesium DV = 400 mg. for men, 310 for women.

Serving Size	Milligrams	% DV
Almonds, dry roasted, 1 ounce	80	20%
Spinach, boiled, ½ cup	78	20
Cashews, dry roasted, 1 ounce	74	19
Pumpkin Seeds, 1 ounce	74	19
Peanuts, oil roasted, ¼ cup	63	16
Cereal, shredded wheat, 2 biscuits	61	15
Soymilk, plain or vanilla, 1 cup	61	15
Black beans, cooked, ½ cup	60	15
Edamame, shelled, cooked, ½ cup	50	13
Peanut butter, smooth, 2 tablespoons	49	12
Bread, whole wheat, 2 slices	46	12
Avocado, cubed, 1 cup	44	11
Potato, baked with skin, 3.5 ounces	43	11
Rice, brown, cooked, ½ cup	42	11
Yogurt, plain, low fat, 8 ounces	42	11

Serving Size	Milligrams	% DV
Breakfast cereals, fortified 10% of DV	40	10
Oatmeal, instant, 1 packet	36	9
Kidney beans, canned, ½ cup	35	9
Banana, 1 medium	32	8
Salmon, Atlantic, farmed, 3 ounces	26	7

These are some of the main food sources of magnesium, this nutrient appears in many other foods at lower concentrations. Dark chocolate is good although you'd have to consume a full 100 gram bar to get 176 mg. of magnesium!

Appendix B (cont.)

2. Zinc DV = 15mg.

Serving Size	Milligrams	% DV
Oysters, cooked, 3 ounces	74	493%
Beef chuck roast, braised, 3 ounces	7	47
Crab, Alaska king, cooked, 3 ounces	6.5	43
Beef patty, broiled, 3 ounces	5.3	35
Breakfast cereal, fortified 25% DV	3.8	25
Lobster, cooked, 3 ounces	3.4	23
Pork chop, loin, cooked, 3 ounces	2.9	19
Baked beans, canned, ½ cup	2.9	19
Chicken, dark meat, cooked, 3 ounces	2.4	16
Yogurt, fruit, low fat, 8 ounces	1.7	11
Cashews, dry roasted, 1 ounce	1.6	11
Chickpeas, cooked, ½ cup	1.3	9
Cheese, Swiss, 1 ounce	1.2	8
Oatmeal, instant, plain,1 packet	1.1	7
Milk, low-fat or non fat, 1 cup	1	7
Almonds, dry roasted, 1 ounce	0.9	6
Kidney beans, cooked, ½ cup	0.9	6
Chicken breast, roasted, skin removed, ½ breast	0.9	6
Cheddar cheese or mozzarella, 1 ounce	0.9	6

These are some of the main food sources of zinc, this nutrient appears in many other foods at lower concentrations.

Appendix B (cont.)

3. Calcium DV = 1,000 mg.

Serving Size	Milligrams	% DV
Yogurt, plain, low fat, 8 ounces	415	42%
Mozzarella, part skim, 1.5 ounces	333	33
Sardines, canned 3 ounces	325	33
Cheddar cheese, 1.5 ounces	307	31
Milk, nonfat, 8 ounces**	299	30
Soymilk, calcium-fortified, 8 ounces	299	30
Milk, (2% milk fat), 8 ounces	293	29
Milk, whole (3.25% milk fat), 8 ounces	276	28
Orange juice, calcium-fortified, 6 ozs.	261	26
Tofu, with calcium sulfate, ½ cup	253	25
Salmon, canned, with bone, 3 ounces	181	18
Cottage cheese, 1% milk fat, 1 cup	138	14
Cereal, calcium-fortified, 1 cup	100–1,000	10–100
Frozen yogurt, vanilla, ½ cup	103	10
Turnip greens, fresh, boiled, ½ cup	99	10
Kale, raw, chopped, 1 cup	100	10
Kale, fresh, cooked, 1 cup	94	9
Ice cream, vanilla, ½ cup	84	8

Appendix B (cont.)

4. Potassium DV = 4,700 mg

Serving Size	Milligrams	% DV
Beet Greens, 1 cup	1309	37%
Avocado, whole	1068	30
Sweet Potato, I medium size	952	27
Potato, I medium size	925	26
Acorn Squash	899	26
Spinach, 1 cup	839	24
Dried Apricots 1/2 cup	755	22
Coconut Water	600	17
Yogurt, 1 cup	579	15
White Beans, 1 cup	502	15
Mushrooms, 1 cup	428	12
Banana, 1 large	422	12

Appendix B (cont.)

5. Vitamin A DV = 5,000 International Units (IU's.)

Serving size	IU per serving	Percent DV
Sweet potato, baked in skin, 1 whole	28,058	561
Beef liver, pan fried, 3 ounces	22,175	444
Spinach, frozen, boiled, ½ cup	11,458	229
Carrots, raw, ½ cup	9,189	184
Pumpkin pie, 1 piece	3,743	249
Cantaloupe, raw, ½ cup	2,706	54
Peppers, sweet, red, raw, ½ cup	2,332	47
Mangos, raw, 1 whole	2,240	45
Black-eyed peas (cowpeas), boiled, 1 cup	1,305	26
Apricots, dried, sulfured, 10 halves	1,261	25
Broccoli, boiled, ½ cup	1,208	24
Ice cream, French vanilla, 1 cup	1,014	20
Cheese, ricotta, part skim, 1 cup	945	19
Tomato juice, canned, ¾ cup	821	16
Herring, Atlantic, pickled, 3 ounces	731	15

Appendix B (cont.)

6. Vitamin C DV = 90 mg

Serving Size	Milligrams	% DV
Red pepper, sweet, raw, ½ cup	95	158%
Orange juice, ¾ cup	93	155
Orange, 1 medium	70	117
Grapefruit juice, ¾ cup	70	117
Kiwifruit, 1 medium	64	107
Green pepper, sweet, raw, ½ cup	60	100
Broccoli, cooked, ½ cup	51	85
Strawberries, fresh, sliced, ½ cup	49	82
Brussels sprouts, cooked, ½ cup	48	80
Grapefruit, ½ medium	39	65
Broccoli, raw, ½ cup	39	65
Tomato juice, ¾ cup	33	55
Cantaloupe, ½ cup	29	48
Cabbage, cooked, ½ cup	28	47
Cauliflower, raw, ½ cup	26	43
Potato, baked, 1 medium	17	28
Tomato, raw, 1 medium	17	28

Appendix B (cont.)

7. Vitamin D DV = 400 IU's

Serving Size	IU's	% DV
Cod liver oil, 1 tablespoon	1,360	340%
Swordfish, cooked, 3 ounces	566	142
Salmon (sockeye), cooked, 3 ounces	447	112
Tuna fish, canned in water, 3 ounces	154	39
Orange juice fortified vitamin D, 1 cup	137	34
Milk, 1 cup	115-124	29-31
Yogurt, fortified with 20% DV 6 ozs	80	20
Margarine, fortified, 1 tablespoon	60	15
Sardines, canned in oil, 2 sardines	46	12
Liver, beef, cooked, 3 ounces	42	11
Egg, 1 large (vitamin D is in the yolk)	41	10
Ready-to-eat cereal, fortified with D	40	10

Appendix B (cont.)

8. Vitamin E DV = 30 IU's

Serving Size	IU's	% DV
Wheat germ oil, 1 tablespoon	20.3	100%
Sunflower seeds, dry roasted, 1 ounce	7.4	37
Almonds, dry roasted, 1 ounce	6.8	34
Sunflower oil, 1 tablespoon	5.6	28
Safflower oil, 1 tablespoon	4.6	25
Hazelnuts, dry roasted, 1 ounce	4.3	22
Peanut butter, 2 tablespoons	2.9	15
Peanuts, dry roasted, 1 ounce	2.2	11
Corn oil, 1 tablespoon	1.9	10
Spinach, boiled, ½ cup	1.9	10
Broccoli, chopped, boiled, ½ cup	1.2	6
Soybean oil, 1 tablespoon	1.1	6
Kiwifruit, 1 medium	1.1	6

Appendix B (cont.)

9. Folic Acid - Vitamin B9 400 micrograms (mcg)

Serving Size	mcg	% DV
Beef liver, braised, 3 ounces	215	54%
Spinach, boiled, ½ cup	131	33
Black-eyed peas boiled, ½ cup	105	26
Breakfast cereals, fortified 25% DV	100	25
Rice, white, cooked, ½ cup	90	23
Asparagus, boiled, 4 spears	89	22
Spaghetti, cooked, enriched, ½ cup†	83	21
Brussels sprouts, frozen, boiled, ½ cup	78	20
Lettuce, romaine, shredded, 1 cup	64	16
Avocado, raw, sliced, ½ cup	59	15
Spinach, raw, 1 cup	58	15
Broccoli, chopped, cooked, ½ cup	52	13
Mustard greens, ½ cup	52	13
Green peas, frozen, boiled, ½ cup	47	12
Kidney beans, canned, ½ cup	46	12
Bread, white, 1 slice†	43	11
Peanuts, dry roasted, 1 ounce	41	10
Wheat germ, 2 tablespoons	40	10
Tomato juice, canned, ¾ cup	36	9

Serving Size	mcg	% DV
Crab, Dungeness, 3 ounces	36	9
Orange juice, ¾ cup	35	9

APPENDIX C - Healthy Recipe Ideas

These are just some samples of the dishes my wife and I prepare on a regular basis. They are not meant to be recipes in the strict sense, because there are no weights and measures included. Although some of these dishes may seem odd I urge you to try them - they are all delicious.

1. Breakfast

Morning Drink
We have this drink every morning before eating any food. Hot water with a little freshly squeezed lemon juice and a tablespoon of organic raw apple cider vinegar. I add a little raw honey to sweeten it up.

Why is this healthy?
Drinking hot water and lemon before you have breakfast is a recommended tonic for helping your digestive system to function better. It's also a good energizer first thing in the morning. In fact there are numerous benefits claimed by proponents of this drink, but I'm not sure they're all true! Bottom line - it works for me and I wouldn't start my day without it.

We always have coffee with the following breakfast meals.

Toast & Cheese with Fruit:
We usually have sprouted grain bread, or gluten-free bread for the toast - 1 slice each We'll add some pieces of cheddar cheese, normally the aged variety. We like to have this with sliced strawberries, or blueberries or other fruit depending on the season. We'll usually have some banana as well. To finish off we'll have a piece of the toast with natural peanut butter.

Why is this healthy?
This is a fairly light meal and is easy to digest. Although cheese contains saturated fat, a small

amount is OK and provides protein. Berries are a great food for all kinds of reasons and should be included in your daily diet. Sprouted grain bread is easier to digest and the body absorbs more of the nutrients than it would from regular whole grain bread. Natural peanut butter contains just the peanuts -no added oils or salt. We keep the peanut butter in the fridge to thicken it up, making it easier to spread.

Boiled Eggs

One of my favorites - this is one or two soft boiled eggs (usually takes 5 minutes in boiling water), eaten from a traditional egg cup. Accompanied with a slice of toast using sprouted grain, or gluten-free bread. We'll usually have some banana and berries as well.

Why is this healthy?

Eggs are packed with nutrients and make a great meal for starting the day. As I said above, the fruit provides many healthy benefits and the sprouted whole grain toast is easy on the digestion.

Oats

You can prepare these in several ways, but I use a very basic approach. I pour 1 cup of boiling water onto 1/2 cup of organic rolled oats (not the instant kind) and mix this up after it stands for a minute or so. Then I add some raisins and fruit, like berries and banana slices and it's ready to go! Believe me - this tastes much better than it sounds...

Why is this healthy?

After my description above you might well be asking yourself this question! Oats however have so many benefits it would take a page or two to describe them all in detail. They contain several essential nutrients, including magnesium and manganese which is necessary for good bone health. Eating oats reduces cholesterol levels in the blood and is good for your cardiovascular system. It can also help reduce your risk of developing diabetes. Need I go on - buy some today!

Cold Cereal

Now here's a tricky one - most of the popular breakfast cereals on supermarket shelves are not as healthy as they claim. Not only do they include added synthetic nutrients, many of them are often loaded with sugar. So read the label before buying!

We usually have something basic like All Bran or Muesli, with milk or almond milk and a fresh fruit topping like strawberries or blueberries.

Why is this healthy?

All Bran is a good source of fiber and a typical serving will have about 50% of the recommended daily allowance. Muesli has plenty of anti-oxidants and protein. It usually contains less added sugar than other cereals. The milk is a good source of protein, although almond milk has much less.

2. Lunch

Soup

A great winter favorite, we usually have vegetarian or chicken. We normally have home-made because the canned variety is often high in salt content and may contain the chemical BPA (Bisphenol A).

Why is this healthy?

Soup contains plenty of vegetables which are good for you (if you stay away from the 'cream of...' ones). Soup is also filling and will keep your satisfied through the afternoon. It's also a great comfort food.

Juice

In the warmer weather my wife and I often enjoy a juice made of a mix of vegetables and fruit. We use the 'Magic Bullet' juicer because it's more of a blender than a juice extractor and so retains the fiber part of the fruit and veggies. We accompany the juice with some bread or crackers and a hummus or black bean dip, or cheese.

Why is this healthy?
Fruit and vegetables are full of nutrients and in liquid form are more easily absorbed by the body. Juicing is a great way to get some of the recommended 6 - 8 daily servings of these food groups. Also hummus and black bean dip add protein to balance the meal.

Yogurt and cottage cheese with fruit
This is an easy one to prepare - just mix two or thee tablespoons of plain yogurt with some cottage cheese to your taste. Add some fruit such as berries, banana, kiwi etc. We often add a little flax seed and pumpkin seeds also. You can accompany this with toast (preferably sprouted grain or sourdough) and a nut butter.

Why is this healthy?
All of the above ingredients have good nutritional value. Yogurt and some types of cottage cheese are fermented which helps you maintain a healthy gut and immune system. Berries and fruit of course have many benefits as we discussed in the Nutrition section.

Sardines on Toast
You may not care for the taste of sardines but they are really good for you. We usually have them on toast along with some tomato and onion. You can spread the toast with mustard for extra flavor.

Why is this healthy?
Sardines contain a good amount of omeg-3 fatty acid as well as important vitamins and minerals (vitamins B12 & D, calcium, potassium and more). Sardines are also wild caught, not farmed.

3. Dinner

Roast chicken with Baked Sweet Potato

This is one of our favorites, we often go to the local market to get a chicken raised in free-run environment without antibiotics. It costs a little more but I think it's worth the extra. We use sweet potatoes to roast (or just regular ones if we don't have them). For vegetables we'll do broccoli, or green beans. This is a fairly basic dish but who doesn't like roast chicken?

Why is this healthy?

Providing it has been properly raised chicken is a good source of healthy protein; it contains all the essential amino acids The white meat has less fat than the dark but is not quite as tasty (don't eat the skin!). It's an important source of B3 and B6 as well as other vitamins and minerals.

Sweet potato is well know for its many healthy qualities. It contains many important nutrients including vitamins A and C and vitamins and minerals.

♥ Health Hint

A boiled sweet potato has a much lower glycemic index than the baked version, so if you want to improve this meal use the boiled version. A lower glycemic index means it has less impact on your blood sugar level.

Stuffed Portobello Mushrooms

This is a very tasty vegetarian (or vegan if you omit the cheese) meal. After baking the mushrooms for fifteen minutes add a mix of sauteed vegetables like tomato, onion, garlic and beans, top with cheese and bake some more. We accompany this with boiled red potatoes and broccoli.

Why is this healthy?

Mushrooms of all kinds contain lots of nutrients and the Portobello variety are no exception. They have the powerful anti-oxidant selenium and other minerals like iron, copper, niacin, potassium and phosphorous. The mushroom along with the beans and cheese provide the protein for this meal.

Grilled or Baked Salmon

We either bake the salmon with a pecan topping in the oven or simply barbecue it. It does need care on the BBQ because it sticks very easily to the grill. Either way this is a delicious meal when the salmon is cooked just right. Asparagus and potatoes go well with the salmon, or you can use rice instead of the potatoes.

Why is this healthy?

Salmon is a good source of protein and also the fatty acid Omega-3, as well as other important nutrients like selenium, astaxanthin, vitamin B and potassium. The wild-caught variety is better than farm-raised. Asparagus is also very beneficial and has antioxidant and anti-inflammatory properties. It is reputed to be good for your heart, digestion and bones.

Greek Salad

What - just salad for dinner? Actually we love this meal in summertime. In addition to the basic mixed greens our version of a Greek salad contains lots of vegetables like onion, tomato, green and red peppers, cucumber etc. We use an Olive oil dressing and add black olives and Feta cheese. We like to enjoy this with a multi-grain Ciabatta baguette and a glass of red wine!

APPENDIX D - Facts On Fats & Oils

The table below has a list of commonly used fats and oils. It's arranged in alphabetical order so you can easily check on a particular oil

Notes:

1. Most oils and fats are a mix of monounsaturated, polyunsaturated and saturated fats. The 'Type' column indicates the predominant one.

2. Polyunsaturated oils are unstable when heated,

3. Oils made from seeds and vegetable sources should be cold pressed (or expeller pressed).

4. The ♥ indicates the healthiest choices for each oil or fat.

5. The 💀 means unhealthy! Try to stay away from using these or eating foods cooked with them.

6. The 'Cooking?' column indicates whether the oil/fat can be used for cooking.

Name	Type / sources	Cooking?	Comments
♥ Avocado Oil	Monounsaturated	Yes	Avocados are very nutritious and the oil contains similar health benefits.
Butter	Saturated	Yes	This is one of the few animal-based fats in this table.
Canola Oil	Monounsaturated. made from genetically modified rapeseeds		Some health experts say that Canola oil is not as healthy as its producers claim
Coconut oil	Saturated	Yes	Good for cooking. Use sparingly - the organic unrefined kind is best.

Name	Type / sources	Cooking?	Comments
☠ Corn Oil	Polyunsaturated	No	Breaks down with heat, may increase your risk of coronary heart disease. Very high in omega-6 fats
Flaxseed oil	Polyunsaturated	No	This is another healthy oil when not heated.
Grape seed oil	Polyunsaturated	No	Breaks down with heat. High in omega-6 fats
♥ Hemp Seed Oil	Polyunsaturated	Low heat	Contains healthy nutrients like vitamin E and carotene. Good ratio of omega-6 to omega-3 fatty acids. Store the unrefined version in a dark bottle in the refrigerator.
☠ Hydrogenated Oil	General category of vegetable and seed oils to which hydrogen is added	No	Contains trans-fats
Lard	Monounsaturated 50% and 40% saturated fats. Usually from pork fat	Yes	Surprisingly not as unhealthy as you might think. However it is animal based and I don't use it.
Margarine	Generally a mix of mono & polyunsaturated mix of fats	No	This has been a controversial alternative to butter for years. I don't use it.
♥ Olive Oil	Monounsaturated	Low heat	One of the healthiest oils. Great for salads and low heat cooking. Make sure to buy the authentic cold pressed oil.
Palm Kernel Oil	High in Saturated fat	Yes	Often used in commercial cooking

Name	Type / sources	Cooking?	Comments
Palm Oil	Mix of saturated and unsaturated plus a small amount of polyunsaturated fat	Yes	Less fat than butter and can be used for cooking
Peanut oil	Monounsaturated	Yes	Good for high heat cooking but it is high in omega-6.
Safflower Oil	Monounsaturated		Nutritious, but high in omega-6
♥ Sesame Seed Oil	Unsaturated with some saturated fat	Yes	Has many health benefits
☠ Shortening	Saturated	Yes	Highly processed and may contain trans-fats
Soybean oil	Polyunsaturated, monounsaturated and saturated	Low heat	Look for organic, non-hydrogenated.
Sunflower Oil	Mostly poly- and monounsaturated fats	Yes if refined.	This comes in different varieties. Unrefined is better but not for cooking
Vegetable Oil	Can contain both unsaturated and saturated fats	Yes	General term for oil extracted from various fruits, seeds, grains and nuts
♥ Walnut Oil	polyunsaturated with some monounsaturated and saturated fats	Lower heat	Good source of anti-oxidants and omega-3 fatty acid. Add it to salad dressings

APPENDIX E - Morning Stretches

This is the morning wake-up routine I've been doing for over twenty years...

It really helps me limber up and helps get rid of the muscle stiffness I often feel after just getting out of bed.

These exercises should be done gently - you've just got up and your muscle flexibility is restricted

1. Overhead Stretch

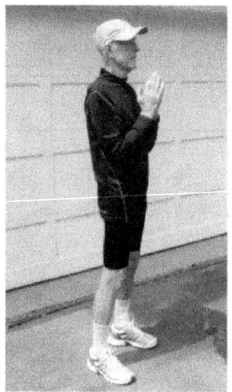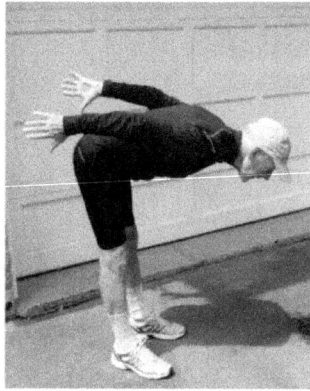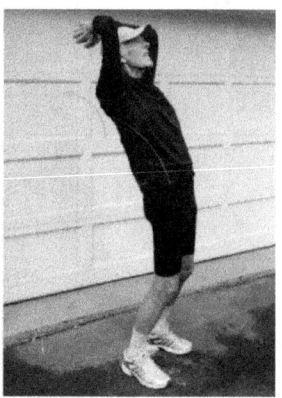

Start with legs apart and hands together as shown. Bend forward from the waist and extend your arms straight out behind you. Breathe out as you are doing this. Then raise your arms above your head as you bend backwards. Breathe in. Return to the start and repeat. I usually do three or four repetitions.

2. Side Stretch

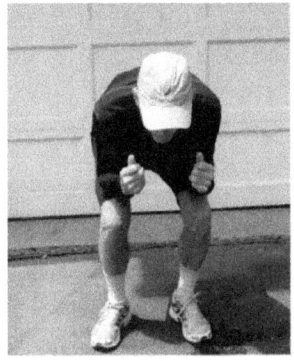 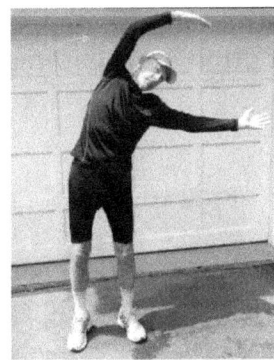 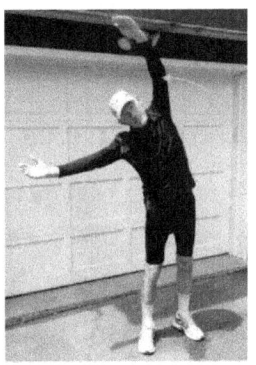

Bend the legs with arms raised and elbows just touching the top of the knees. Straighten up and extend your arms as shown, as you lean your upper body to the left side, breathing in as you do this. Then slowly return to the starting position breathing out as you go. Then do the same thing but on your right side. You can do three or four repetitions of the full movement.

3. Head Rotation

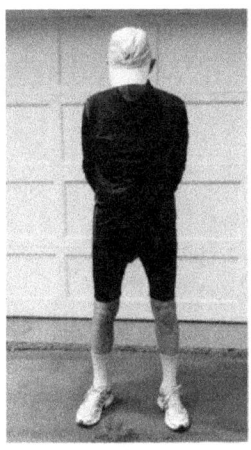 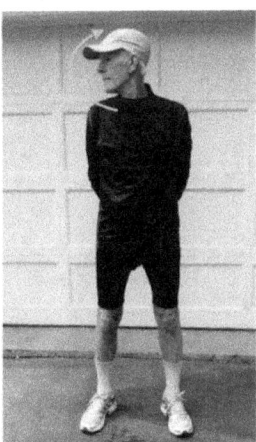 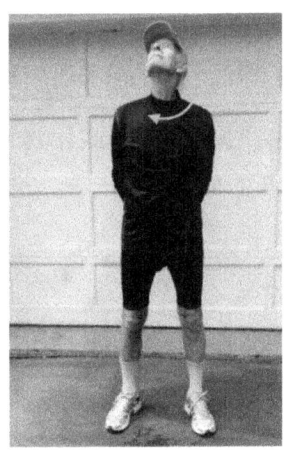

Breathe out with you head and neck down. Straighten the neck and head to look straight in front. Slowly rotate the head to the left in a circular motion three or four times, breathing in as you go. Return to the starting position with the head down and breathe out completely. Repeat the head rotation, only this time rotate the head to the right and return to starting position. This completes this exercise.

4. Arm Circles

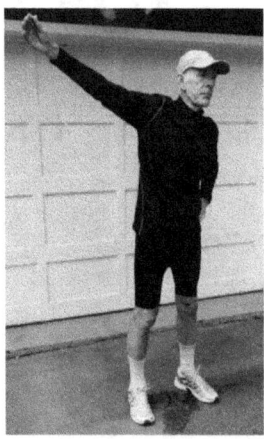
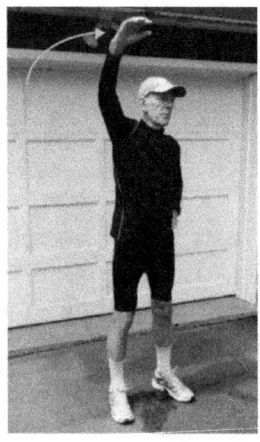
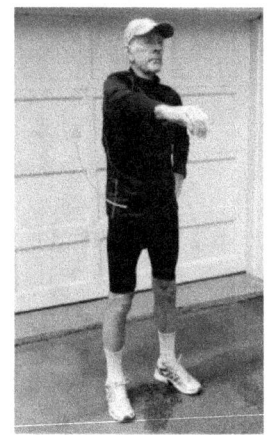

A good warm-up exercise for the shoulders, arms, chest, and back. Standing straight, rotate the right arm in forward circles about 10 times, breathing normally. Then rotate the arm backwards, again about 10 rotations. Now repeat the exercise with the left arm.

5. Core Rotation

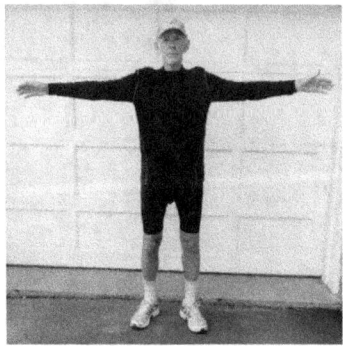
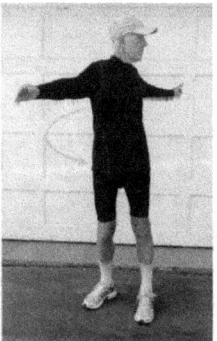
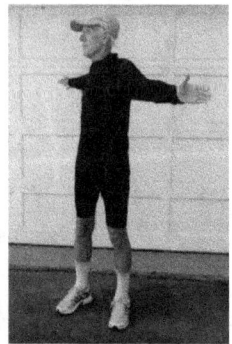

This helps keep flexibility in your core muscles and works your lower spine. Stand straight with arms straight out to the side, then slowly turn the upper torso to the left breathing in. Then return to the starting position breathing out completely. Continue the motion turning to the right and breathing in again. Do half a dozen reps.

6. Hip rotation

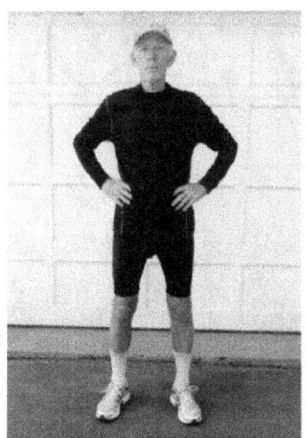 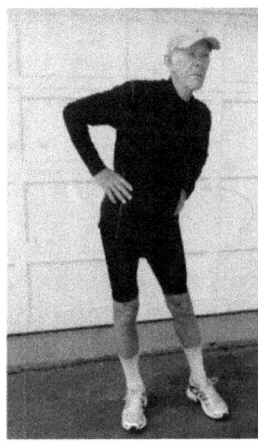 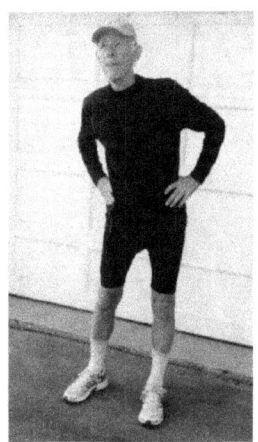

Start with your hand on hips, looking straight ahead. Then rotate the pelvis leftwards in a circular motion. Do this about six or more times as you breathe in. Then reverse the motion going to the right as you slowly breathe out.

7. Leg & Arm Stretch

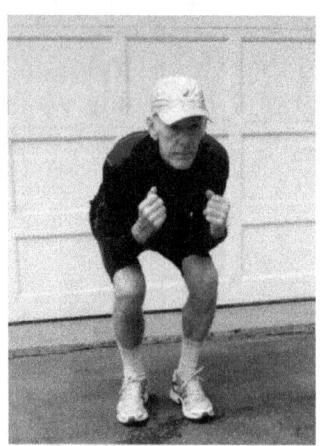 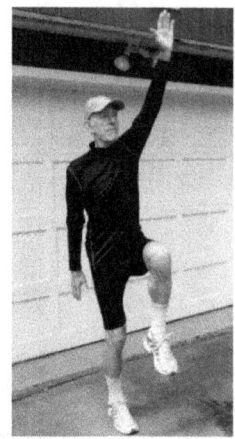 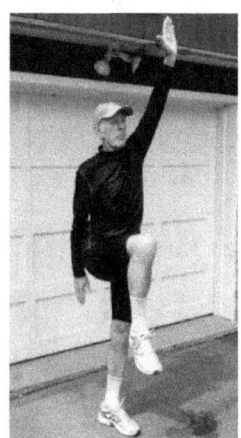

This is good for improving your balance. With your feet a few inches apart, Start in the position shown with elbows on knees. Raise the left arm above your head and lift your left leg so the knee is horizontal. A variation of this is to use the alternate arm and leg as shown in the third picture, so your left arm would be raised while you stand on your left leg and raise the right knee.

Stand for a few seconds (or more!) on the one leg, breathing in. Then lower your arm and leg, breathing out. Repeat with the right side so you're standing on your other leg. Two or three reps. will do.

8. Hamstring Stretch

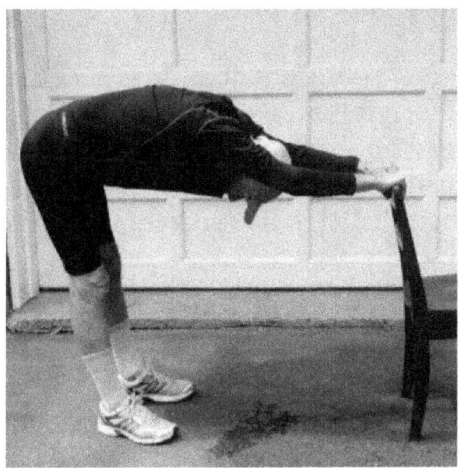 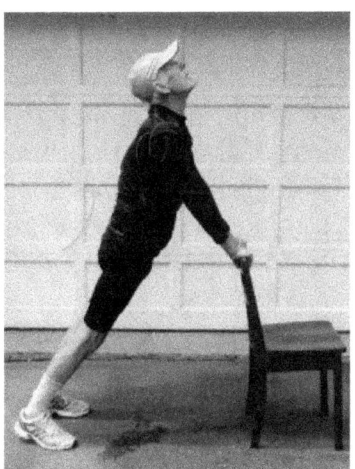

This is good for the muscles in the back of your legs, all the way from the lower spine through the hamstrings and calves. You need a support like a table or desk for this one. With your hands out in front on the edge of the table bend over so that your back is almost horizontal. Breathe out as you do this. Then still holding on, raise your upper body until it is bending backwards. Breathe in as you do this. Don't strain.

Repeat four or five times.

REFERENCES

Note: The following references represent just some of the research I did while writing 'Forty plus Thirty' but they cover most of the main points I mention in the book. I've included a website URL so you can read each full article if you wish. To make this easier I have included this list of references on the Forty plus Thirty website:

http://fortyplusthirty.com/

All you have to do is go to the 'References' page and click the link on each reference.

Section 1. Health

1-1 National Health Council, Report on Chronic Diseases
http://www.nationalhealthcouncil.org/sites/default/files/N HC_Files/Pdf_Files/AboutChronicDisease.pdf

1-2 Centers for Disease Control CDC; Chronic Disease Overview
https://www.cdc.gov/chronicdisease/overview/index.htm

1-3 World Health Organization; Life Expectancy Ranking by Country,
https://en.wikipedia.org/wiki/List_of_countries_by_life_ex pectancy

1-4 CDC Assessing Your Weight
https://www.cdc.gov/healthyweight/assessing/index.html

1-5 Medical Daily; The Reason Why Americans Have Lower Life Expectancy Than Other High-Income Countries explains the impact of injury-related deaths
https://www.medicaldaily.com/life-expectancy-injury-high-income-countries-372832

1-6 CDC National Center for Health Statistics; <u>Mortality in the United States, 2016</u>
https://www.cdc.gov/nchs/products/databriefs/db293.htm

1-7 7 Drew University; <u>Elements of Wellness</u>
https://www.drew.edu/CampusRec/wellness/7-elements-of-wellness

1-8 World Health Organization; <u>Mental health: a state of well-being</u>
http://www.who.int/features/factfiles/mental_health/en/

1-9 WebMD; <u>Genes vs. Lifestyle: What Matters Most for Health?</u>
https://www.webmd.com/healthy-aging/features/genes-or-lifestyle

1-10 Dr. Mercola; <u>Top Ten Ways the American Health Care System Fails</u>
https://articles.mercola.com/sites/articles/archive/2014/03/15/bad-american-health-care-system.aspx

1-11 Journal of the Royal Society of Medicine, Judith Rowbotham & Paul Clayton; <u>Victorian consumption patterns and their health benefits</u>
https://www.ncbi.nlm.nih.gov/pmc/articles/PMC2587384/

2 Nutrition

2-1 James Beckerman, M.D.; <u>Eat a salad every day</u> Dr. Beckerman is author of The Flex Diet: Design-Your-Own Weight Loss Plan (Simon & Schuster, 2010.

2-2 American Institute for Cancer Research; <u>Going Cuckoo for Color</u>
http://www.aicr.org/new-american-plate/nap-challenge/week-9.html?_ga=2.170925024.1718068929.1526990657-272663770.1526990654

2-3 Ying Bao, M.D. Sc.D; Study: Association of Nut Consumption with Total and Cause-Specific Mortality published in New England Journal of Medicine
http://www.nejm.org/doi/full/10.1056/NEJMoa1307352

2-4 Toby Amidor, MS, RD, CDN; Are You Eating Enough Fish? Sept. 4, 2015
http://health.usnews.com/health-news/blogs/eat-run/2015/09/04/are-you-eating-enough-fish

2-5 a) The American Cancer Institute; Recommendations for Cancer Prevention
http://www.aicr.org/reduce-your-cancer-risk/recommendations-for-cancer-prevention/recommendations_05_red_meat.html?_ga=1.47099361.775236235.1478867660

b) Mayo Clinic Staff, Meatless meals; The benefits of eating less meat
http://www.mayoclinic.org/healthy-lifestyle/nutrition-and-healthy-eating/in-depth/meatless-meals/art-20048193?pg=2

2-6 Mayo Clinic Staff; Water: How much should you drink every day?
http://www.mayoclinic.org/healthy-lifestyle/nutrition-and-healthy-eating/in-depth/water/art-20044256

2-7 Lorien E. Urban, PHD; Study: Energy Contents of Frequently Ordered Restaurant Meals... April 2016
http://www.andjrnl.org//S2212-26721501736-0/abstract

2-8 Rachel K. Johnson, PhD, et al, Study: Dietary Sugars Intake and Cardiovascular Health A Scientific Statement From the American Heart Association. Sept. 15, 2009
http://circ.ahajournals.org/content/circulationaha/120/11/1011.full.pdf

2-9 National Public Radio (NPR); <u>Food As Medicine: It's Not Just A Fringe Idea Anymore,</u> Jan. 17, 2017
https://www.npr.org/sections/thesalt/2017/01/17/5095208
95/food-as-medicine-it-s-not-just-a-fringe-idea-anymore

2-10 Berkley Wellness, University of California; <u>Is High-Fructose Corn Syrup Worse Than Regular Sugar?</u>
http://www.berkeleywellness.com/healthy-eating/nutrition/article/high-fructose-corn-syrup-worse-regular-sugar

2-11 American Institute for Cancer Research; <u>Processed foods, calories and nutrients: Americans' alarming diet.</u> June 13, 2017
http://blog.aicr.org/2017/06/13/processed-foods-calories-and-nutrients-americans-alarming-diet/

2-12 SFGate; <u>Does the Body Process Fruit Sugars the Same Way That It Does Refined Sugar?</u>
http://healthyeating.sfgate.com/body-process-fruit-sugars-same-way-refined-sugar-8174.html

2-13 EUFIC - The European Food Information Council; <u>8 Facts on Fats (Q&A)</u>
http://www.eufic.org/en/whats-in-food/article/8-facts-on-fats

2-14 University Health News; <u>Omega-6 vs. Omega-3 Fatty Acids: What You Should Know</u>
https://universityhealthnews.com/daily/nutrition/omega-6-vs-omega-3-fatty-acids/

2-15 Scientific World Journal, Margaret E. Sears; <u>Chelation: Harnessing and Enhancing Heavy Metal Detoxification—A Review</u>
https://www.ncbi.nlm.nih.gov/pmc/articles/PMC3654245/

2-16 Healthline; <u>Pastured vs Omega-3 vs Conventional Eggs — What's the Difference?</u>

https://www.healthline.com/nutrition/pastured-vs-omega-3-vs-conventional-eggs - modal-close

2-17 BBC News; Seven-a-day fruit and veg 'saves lives
http://www.bbc.com/news/health-26818377

2-18 National Institute of Health, Naghma Khan and Hasan Mukhtar; Tea and Health: Studies in Humans
https://www.ncbi.nlm.nih.gov/pmc/articles/PMC4055352/

2-19 American Institute for Cancer Research; The Spices of Cancer Prevention
http://www.aicr.org/cancer-research-update/august_21_2013/CRU_spices_cancer_prevention.html?_ga=2.167050430.1076280699.1525180797-1473894658.1525180797

2-20   Institute of Environmental Medicine, Karolinska Institutet, Stockholm, A. Wolk; Potential health hazards of eating red meat
https://onlinelibrary.wiley.com/doi/pdf/10.1111/joim.12543

2-21 Stanford Medical News Center; Study shows link between canned food, exposure to hormone-disrupting chemical
https://med.stanford.edu/news/all-news/2016/06/link-between-canned-food-exposure-to-hormone-disrupting-chemical.html

2-22 American Heart Association; Saturated Fat
https://healthyforgood.heart.org/eat-smart/articles/saturated-fats

2-23 Havard Health Blog, Howard LeWine, M.D.; Fish oil: friend or foe?
https://www.health.harvard.edu/blog/fish-oil-friend-or-foe-201307126467

2-24 7 Prevention Magazine; 7 Essential Nutrients You're Missing
https://www.prevention.com/food/healthy-eating-tips/7-essential-nutrients-healthy-diet

3. Exercise

3-1 Prevention Magazine; Which One's More Important: Diet Or Exercise?
https://www.prevention.com/weight-loss/diet-vs-exercise

3-2 American Heart Association; Recommendations for Physical Activity in Adults February 2014
http://www.heart.org/HEARTORG/HealthyLiving/Physical Activity/FitnessBasics/American-Heart-Association-Recommendations-for-Physical-Activity-in-Adults_UCM_307976_Article.jsp - .WudgqooY7v8

3-3 Neville Owen, PhD et al. Sedentary Behavior: Emerging Evidence for a New Health Risk 2010

https://www.ncbi.nlm.nih.gov/pmc/articles/PMC2996155/

3-4 James A. Levine, M.D., Ph.D.; What are the risks of sitting too much?
http://www.mayoclinic.org/healthy-lifestyle/adult-health/expert-answers/sitting/faq-20058005

3-5 JACC: Clinical Electrophysiology Atrial Fibrillation in Athletes
http://electrophysiology.onlinejacc.org/content/3/9/921

3-6 Livestrong.com; Does Cardio Produce Free Radicals?
https://www.livestrong.com/article/479238-does-cardio-produce-free-radicals/

3-7 National Public Radio, Cosmos and culture; Running And Your Heart: Is There A 'Too Much?'
https://www.npr.org/sections/13.7/2017/07/26/539458731/running-and-your-heart-is-there-a-too-much

3-8 Health.com; <u>What to Know About Rhabdomyolysis, the Potentially Fatal Condition Caused by Extreme Exercise</u>
http://www.health.com/fitness/rhabdomyolysis

4. Power of The Mind

4-1 Wikipedia; <u>Neuroplasticity</u>
https://en.wikipedia.org/wiki/Neuroplasticity

4-2 National Institute for Health; <u>Neuroplasticity and Clinical Practice: Building Brain Power for Health</u>
https://www.ncbi.nlm.nih.gov/pmc/articles/PMC4960264/

4-3 Tonic; <u>Elite Athletes Visualize Their Obstacles to Push Past Them</u>
https://tonic.vice.com/en_us/article/bjyemm/can-visualization-help-athletes

4-4 Health Central.com; <u>Getting to Know Your 5 Essential Brain Chemicals</u>
https://www.healthcentral.com/slideshow/getting-to-know-your-5-essential-brain-chemicals

4-5 Mental Health foundation; <u>Physical health and mental health</u>
https://www.mentalhealth.org.uk/a-to-z/p/physical-health-and-mental-health

4-6 National Institute on Aging; <u>How the Aging Brain Affects Thinking</u>
https://www.nia.nih.gov/health/how-aging-brain-affects-thinking

4-7 Fortanasce, <u>Test Your Real Brain Age</u>
http://www.healthybrainmd.com/conditions-treat/test-real-brain-age/

4-8 Harvard Medical School; Regular exercise changes the brain to improve memory, thinking skills
https://www.health.harvard.edu/blog/regular-exercise-changes-brain-improve-memory-thinking-skills-201404097110

4-9 Harvard Medical School; High blood sugar linked to brain shrinkage
https://www.health.harvard.edu/diseases-and-conditions/high-blood-sugar-linked-to-brain-shrinkage

4-10 Harvard Medical School; Eating nuts linked to healthier, longer life
https://www.health.harvard.edu/blog/eating-nuts-linked-to-healthier-longer-life-201311206893

4-11 Psychology Today; Chronic Stress Can Damage Brain Structure and Connectivity
https://www.psychologytoday.com/us/blog/the-athletes-way/201402/chronic-stress-can-damage-brain-structure-and-connectivity

4-12 American Psychological Association; Stress Effects on the Body
http://www.apa.org/helpcenter/stress-body.aspx

4-13 University of California, Irvine Institute for Brain Aging and Dementia; Exercise builds brain health: key roles of growth factor cascades and inflammation
https://pdfs.semanticscholar.org/acba/2db2954f38241bae6261d33c80dedd5d3b86.pdf

4-14 IFL Science; Cigarette Smoke Could Thin Cerebral Cortex
http://www.iflscience.com/health-and-medicine/cigarette-smoke-could-thin-cerebral-cortex/

4-15 Medical News today; Why stress happens and how to manage it https://www.medicalnewstoday.com/articles/145855.php

4-16 Prevention Magazine, Keri Glassman, MS, RD, CDN; 13 Foods That Fight Stress
https://www.prevention.com/mind-body/emotional-health/13-healthy-foods-that-reduce-stress-and-depression

4-17 Mayo Clinic; Exercise and stress: Get moving to manage stress
https://www.mayoclinic.org/healthy-lifestyle/stress-management/in-depth/exercise-and-stress/art-20044469

4-18 Mayo Clinic; Meditation: A simple, fast way to reduce stress
https://www.mayoclinic.org/tests-procedures/meditation/in-depth/meditation/art-20045858

4-19 Health.com; 11 Surprising Health Benefits of Sleep
http://www.health.com/health/gallery/0,,20459221,00.html - curb-inflammation-0

4-20 CBS News; AAA study finds risks of drowsy driving comparable to drunk driving
https://www.cbsnews.com/news/aaa-study-drowsy-driving-dangers-comparable-to-drunk-driving/

4-21 WebMD; Understanding the Side Effects of Sleeping Pills
https://www.webmd.com/sleep-disorders/guide/understanding-the-side-effects-of-sleeping-pills - 1

5. The Inside Story

5-1 Men's Health; 6 Essential Blood Tests You Should Have
https://www.menshealth.com/health/a19538154/6-essential-blood-tests-you-should-have/

5-2 WebMD; What Is a Comprehensive Metabolic Panel?
https://www.webmd.com/a-to-z-guides/comprehensive-metabolic-panel - 1

5-3 University of Leicester, UK; DNA, genes and chromosomes
https://www2.le.ac.uk/projects/vgec/schoolsandcolleges/topics/dnageneschromosomes

5-4 Stanford University, The Tech; People are not as alike as scientists once thought
http://genetics.thetech.org/original_news/news38

5-5 National Humane Genome Research Institute; An Overview of the Human Genome Project
https://www.genome.gov/12011238/an-overview-of-the-human-genome-project/

5-6 The Guardian; Do your genes determine your entire life?
https://www.theguardian.com/science/2015/mar/19/do-your-genes-determine-your-entire-life

5-7 Cancer Research UK; Can cancer be prevented?
http://www.cancerresearchuk.org/about-cancer/causes-of-cancer/can-cancer-be-prevented

6. Live Better, Live Longer

6-1 Merck Manuals; Changes in the Body With Aging
https://www.merckmanuals.com/en-ca/home/older-people%E2%80%99s-health-issues/the-aging-body/changes-in-the-body-with-aging

6-2 YellowPages.ca; A quick guide to aging: what to expect in every decade
https://www.yellowpages.ca/tips/a-quick-guide-to-aging-what-to-expect-in-every-decade/

6-3 Karen Collins, MS, RD, CDN, American Institute for Cancer Research; More Vegetables, More Colors http://www.aicr.org/press/health-features/nutrition-notes/nn-more-vegetables-more-colors.html

6-4 New England Journal of Medicine ,Ying Bao, M.D.; Association of Nut Consumption with Total and Cause-Specific Mortality
http://www.nejm.org/doi/full/10.1056/NEJMoa1307352

6-5 U.S. News, Toby Amidor, MS, RD, CDN; Are You Eating Enough Fish?
http://health.usnews.com/health-news/blogs/eat-run/2015/09/04/are-you-eating-enough-fish

6-6 The American Cancer Institute; Recommendations for Cancer Prevention
http://www.aicr.org/reduce-your-cancer-risk/recommendations-for-cancer-prevention/recommendations_05_red_meat.html?_ga=1.47099361.775236235.1478867660

6-7 Mayo Clinic Staff; Water: How much should you drink every day?
http://www.mayoclinic.org/healthy-lifestyle/nutrition-and-healthy-eating/in-depth/water/art-20044256

6-8 Lorien E. Urban, PHD; Energy Contents of Frequently Ordered Restaurant Meals...
http://www.andjrnl.org/article/S2212-2672(15)01736-0/abstract

6-9 American Heart Association, Rachel K. Johnson, PhD, et al; Dietary Sugars Intake and Cardiovascular Health A Scientific Statement
http://circ.ahajournals.org/content/circulationaha/120/11/1011.full.pdf

6-10 American Heart Association; Recommendations for Physical Activity in Adults http://www.heart.org/HEARTORG/HealthyLiving/Physical Activity/FitnessBasics/American-Heart-Association-Recommendations-for-Physical-Activity-in-Adults_UCM_307976_Article.jsp - .WvGQBY0Y7v8

6-11 National Institute for Health, Neville Owen, PhD et al; Sedentary Behavior: Emerging Evidence for a New Health Risk
https://www.ncbi.nlm.nih.gov/pmc/articles/PMC2996155/

6-12 Mayo clinic, James A. Levine, M.D., Ph.D.; What are the risks of sitting too much?
http://www.mayoclinic.org/healthy-lifestyle/adult-health/expert-answers/sitting/faq-20058005

6-13 American Psychological Association; Stress
http://www.apa.org/topics/stress/

6-14 The Dana Sourcebook of Immunology; The Immune System's Role in Protection
http://www.dana.org/Publications/ReportDetails.aspx?id=44163

6-15 Harvard Health Publications; How to boost your immune system -Tips to fight disease and strengthen immunity http://www.health.harvard.edu/staying-healthy/how-to-boost-your-immune-system

6-16 National Public Radio; Habits: How They Form And How To Break Them
https://www.npr.org/2012/03/05/147192599/habits-how-they-form-and-how-to-break-them

6-17 Fitness Magazine; What Your Gut Says About Your Health
https://www.fitnessmagazine.com/health/digestive-system-health/

6-18 World Health Organization; <u>Q&A on the carcinogenicity of the consumption of red meat and processed meat</u>
http://www.who.int/features/qa/cancer-red-meat/en/

6-19 World Life Expectancy; <u>Sit less and live longer!</u>
http://www.worldlifeexpectancy.com/sit-less-and-live-longer

6-20 The Canadian Heart & Stroke Foundation; <u>Get Healthy Prevention is key</u>
http://www.heartandstroke.ca/get-healthy?gclid=EAIaIQobChMI8-Kby6T72gIVAwxpCh3MbQT8EAAYASAAEgLpL_D_BwE

www.ingramcontent.com/pod-product-compliance
Lightning Source LLC
Chambersburg PA
CBHW060452290526
45791CB00001B/76